VOLUME I of the Network Based Diabetes Care (NBDC) series

EATING AGAINST *the* NETWORK

A CLINICAL FRAMEWORK FOR TYPE 2 DIABETES

Enrique C. Fernández, MD

Published by NBDC Press

Eating Against The Network:
A Clinical Framework for Type 2 Diabetes

First Edition, 2026

Published by NBDC Press

Paperback ISBN: 979-8-9954491-0-2

eBook ISBN: 979-8-9954491-2-6

Medical Disclaimer
This book is intended for general educational and informational purposes only. It is not a substitute for professional medical advice, diagnosis, or treatment, and nothing in it establishes a physician–patient relationship. The information reflects the author's clinical experience and the published science available at the time of writing; medical knowledge evolves, and individual circumstances vary.

Always consult your own physician or a qualified healthcare provider before making any change to your diet, medications, supplements, fasting practices, or exercise routine — particularly if you take glucose-lowering medication such as insulin or a sulfonylurea, for which dietary and fasting changes can cause hypoglycemia. Do not disregard or delay seeking professional medical advice because of something you have read here.

The author and publisher have made reasonable efforts to ensure accuracy but make no warranties as to the completeness or applicability of the contents to any individual. They disclaim any liability, loss, or risk incurred as a direct or indirect consequence of the use or application of any information in this book.

Cover and interior design: Scott Moden

Series Designer, *Network Based Diabetes Care (NBDC):* Scott Moden

Printed in the United States of America

Contents

To my parents,

whose guidance shaped my core,

and to my patients,

who showed me the path.

Preface

Your body is responding to your last meal right now. Not metaphorically. The molecules from what you ate two hours ago are circulating through your bloodstream, binding to receptors, triggering cascades, leaving traces. Some of those traces will be cleared by tomorrow. Others will remain for weeks, for months, for the rest of your life. The chemistry does not pause when you stop thinking about it. It does not ask your permission. It is happening, right now, regardless of whether you are aware of it.

This is the difficult truth at the center of type 2 diabetes. The disease is not, fundamentally, a problem of blood sugar. Blood sugar is a measurement — a useful one, but a downstream one. The actual disease is a network of self-amplifying chemical reactions that begins in the bloodstream and spreads, over years and decades, into the tissues of the kidneys, the eyes, the nerves, the heart, and the brain. Glucose is the trigger. The damage is done by what glucose does next.

I have practiced family medicine in Miami for more than twenty years. In that time I have watched type 2 diabetes do its work on hundreds of patients. I have watched it move slowly in some and aggressively in others. I have watched two patients with identical hemoglobin A1c numbers follow radically different trajectories — one losing kidney function in five years, the other walking into my office a decade later still asymptomatic. I have watched patients who did everything their physicians asked of them progress relentlessly, and patients who made one focused change in their eating reverse course in ways their textbooks said should not be possible.

Those observations did not match the conventional model I was taught. The conventional model says: lower the glucose, prevent the complications. It is not wrong, exactly, but it is incomplete. It treats diabetes as a single variable problem and the body as a passive recipient of pharmacology. What I was seeing in twenty-five years of practice was something else: a network of seven distinct molecular pathways, each amplifying the others, each responsive to specific dietary and behavioral inputs, each with its own time course and its own reversibility. The patients whose disease moved slowly were the ones whose diets, often unintentionally, suppressed multiple pathways at once. The patients whose disease moved quickly were the ones whose diets fed it.

This book is an attempt to describe what I have seen, in language that both physicians and patients can use. It is built around what I call the Network Based Diabetes Care framework, or NBDC: a model that organizes the chemistry of type 2 diabetes into seven interconnected nodes and traces the specific foods, eating patterns, and timing strategies that intervene at each node. The framework is grounded in published biochemistry, in pharmacology I have practiced for two decades, and in the longitudinal observations of a real primary-care cohort. None of it is speculative. All of it is happening, in real time, in the body of every person reading this sentence.

I want to be clear about what this book is not. It is not a diet book in the conventional sense. I will not tell you that one food is forbidden and another is required. I will not promise that eating a particular vegetable will reverse your diabetes. I will not moralize about food choices, because the chemistry does not moralize. Your body is not punishing you for eating a croissant; it is metabolizing the croissant according to laws that operate on every cell, in every person, in exactly the same way. What changes from person to person is not the chemistry. What changes is the cumulative effect of the chemistry over time, and the points at which we choose to intervene.

Knowing this changes things. Not because knowledge prevents disease — sometimes it does, sometimes it doesn't — but because knowledge transforms your relationship to the disease. The patient who understands that the glucose spike from a sugary breakfast will activate inflammatory signaling in their endothelium for the next four hours is a different patient from one who simply feels guilty afterward. The first patient can think about timing, about food sequence, about what to eat with the breakfast to soften the spike. The second patient is trapped in a moral framework that does not match the underlying biology. The chemistry was going to happen either way. Understanding it makes you stronger, because it makes you a participant rather than a passenger.

This book is written for two audiences at once, and I make no apology for that. Physicians will find a clinical framework they can use with their type 2 diabetes patients tomorrow morning. Patients and informed readers will find a guide to the chemistry of their own metabolism — explained at the level of mechanism, not metaphor. The two audiences do not need separate books because they are not, at the level of biology, separate problems. The physician is treating the same network the patient is living inside. The more both of them understand it, the better the conversations between them become.

A note on what comes next. Part I lays out the chemistry — the seven nodes of the damage network and how they interact. Part II works through what food does to each node, with specific recommendations grounded in evidence. Part III translates the chemistry into the numbers patients actually encounter: glycemic load, portion sizes, the practical mathematics of the kitchen. Part IV turns to timing — when you eat, when you fast, how exercise fits in. Part V explores the more recent frontier of polyphenols, supplements, and the surprising discoveries in bitter receptor biology. Part VI puts the framework together into a week of eating against the network, and gives patients language for the conversation with their physicians.

Type 2 diabetes is a chronic disease. It is not generally cured, and I am suspicious of any book that promises otherwise. But the trajectory of a chronic disease is not fixed. The chemistry is going to happen. The question is what you do with the understanding of it.

Enrique C. Fernández, MD, MBA, FAAFP

Miami, Florida

June, 2026

PART I

The Chemistry You Cannot See

Your blood sugar is reacting with your proteins right now. The reaction is slow, cumulative, and largely irreversible. Understanding it changes everything about how you think about food.

Most people with type 2 diabetes receive the same dietary instruction: eat less sugar, reduce carbohydrates, lose weight if you can. The advice is not wrong. But it is incomplete in a way that matters — because it describes *what* to do without explaining *why*. And the why, it turns out, is one of the most compelling stories in all of medicine.

The four chapters of Part I tell that story. They describe what actually happens inside your body when blood sugar stays elevated — not in the vague language of "complications" and "risk factors," but in the specific, molecular, step-by-step chemistry of how glucose damages tissue. The story involves a reaction first described by a French chemist in 1912 who was studying why bread turns brown when toasted. It involves a network of seven interconnected molecular processes that amplify each other. It involves the discovery that cells can write the history of blood sugar exposure into their DNA packaging — a kind of molecular memory that persists for years after blood sugar is normalized.

You do not need a background in chemistry or biology to follow this story. You need only one thing: the willingness to understand your own disease at the level at which it actually operates. Because the physician who understands the chemistry manages it differently than the physician who does not. And the patient who understands it makes different choices — not because they are more disciplined, but because the knowledge itself changes the way the choice feels.

CHAPTER 1

The Reaction That Started at Breakfast

Margaret is fifty-four years old. She has had type 2 diabetes for seven years. On a Tuesday morning in November she eats what she has eaten almost every weekday morning for the past decade: two slices of white toast with strawberry jam and a cup of coffee with two sugars. She takes her metformin with breakfast, as instructed. She checks her blood sugar before eating — 118 mg/dL, acceptable — and heads to work.

By 7:15 in the morning, the glucose from those two slices of toast and that jam is moving through Margaret's intestinal wall and entering her bloodstream. Her blood sugar, which was 118 before breakfast, will peak somewhere around 185 to 210 mg/dL within the next hour — a standard postprandial spike for a person with her degree of insulin resistance.

By 7:20 in the morning — five minutes after the glucose enters her bloodstream — it has begun doing something that no one has ever explained to Margaret and that her physician has never had time to describe. The glucose molecules are reacting with the proteins in her body.

Not metaphorically. Not eventually. Right now, as she drives to work, glucose is chemically bonding to the proteins in her blood vessel walls. It is bonding to the proteins in the tiny filters of her kidneys. It is bonding to the crystallin proteins that give the lenses of her eyes their transparency. It is bonding to the myelin sheath that insulates the nerves in her feet and hands. It is bonding to the collagen that gives her arterial walls their structure and flexibility.

The reaction is silent. It produces no pain, no warning, no signal of any kind that Margaret can detect. It has been happening every morning for seven years — and for the seven to ten years before her diagnosis when her blood sugar was elevated without anyone knowing it. The cumulative products of this reaction are sitting in Margaret's tissues right now, and they will not leave.

This reaction — the non-enzymatic bonding of glucose to protein — is the molecular origin of every complication that diabetes produces. Understanding it is not a medical luxury. It is the foundation of every dietary choice that has the power to slow what is happening in Margaret's tissues.

THE SCIENCE BEHIND THIS

The Maillard Reaction: From Kitchen to Body

In 1912, the French physician and chemist Louis Camille Maillard published a paper describing what happened when he heated amino acids and sugars together in a flask. He observed that the mixture turned yellow, then brown, and eventually produced the characteristic flavors and aromas of cooked food. The browning of bread crust, the searing of a steak, the roasting of coffee beans, the caramelization of onions – all of these involve the Maillard reaction. It is one of the most important reactions in food chemistry and, as it turns out, one of the most important reactions in the pathology of diabetes.[1]

The Maillard reaction begins with a simple chemical event: the free amino group on a protein – typically the epsilon-amino group of lysine or the alpha-amino terminus of the protein chain – reacts with the carbonyl group of a reducing sugar, most commonly glucose. This produces a Schiff base: a loose, reversible chemical bond between the protein and the sugar molecule. At this early stage, the reaction can still go backwards – the glucose can detach from the protein and the protein returns to its original state.

But the Schiff base does not stay as a Schiff base for long. Within hours to days, it undergoes a spontaneous rearrangement called the Amadori rearrangement – a proton transfer that converts the unstable Schiff base into a more stable compound called an Amadori product. The Amadori product is considerably more resistant to reversal than the Schiff base. It can still be partially undone, but it tends to persist. The most familiar example of an Amadori product in medicine is HbA1c – the glycated hemoglobin that your physician measures as the primary indicator of your average blood sugar over the past three months. When your HbA1c is measured, what is being quantified is the amount of Amadori product that has formed on the hemoglobin in your red blood cells.

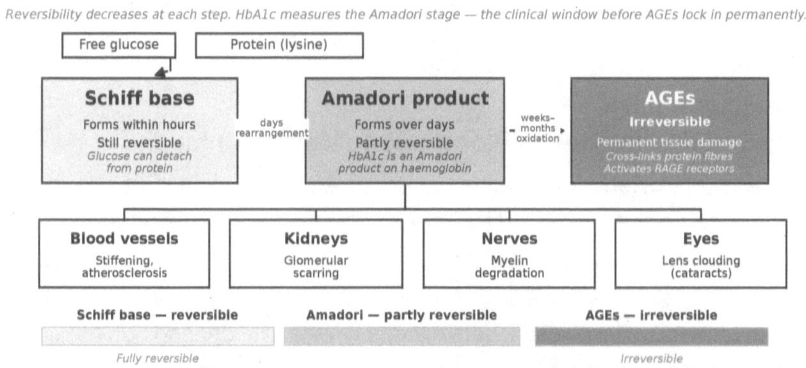

FIGURE 1. The glycation cascade: from Schiff base to Amadori product to AGEs — reversibility decreases at each step.

This is where the reaction's consequences diverge from what happens in a toasted piece of bread. In a kitchen, the Maillard reaction is driven by high heat — 140 to 165 degrees Celsius. At those temperatures, the reaction proceeds rapidly and produces the brown pigments and flavors we associate with cooked food. In the human body, the temperature is only 37 degrees Celsius. The reaction proceeds far more slowly. But the body is not a kitchen, and the proteins in the body are not being discarded after cooking. They are long-lived structures that remain in tissues for months, years, or decades. And over those months and years, the slow Maillard reaction accumulates.

From Amadori Products to Advanced Glycation End-Products[2]

The Amadori product is not the endpoint of the reaction — it is the beginning of a second, more dangerous phase. Over weeks to months, Amadori products undergo further chemical transformations: oxidation, dehydration, condensation with other Amadori products, and cross-linking with neighboring proteins. These reactions produce a diverse family of compounds collectively called Advanced Glycation End-Products, or AGEs.

Unlike the Amadori product, AGEs are essentially irreversible. The chemical cross-links they form between proteins — particularly between collagen fibers in the extracellular matrix — cannot be broken by any enzyme the body produces. Once an AGE has formed, it stays. It accumulates in the long-lived proteins of the body: in the collagen of arterial walls (making them stiffer and less elastic), in the crystallin proteins of the eye lens (making them opaque – the chemical basis of diabetic cataract), in the myelin sheath of peripheral nerves (impeding nerve conduction), in the glomerular basement membrane of the kidney (thickening the filtration barrier), and in the proteins of cardiac muscle (contributing to the diastolic stiffness of the diabetic heart).[3]

The Square Law: Why Small Increases in Blood Sugar Matter So Much

The most important quantitative feature of AGE formation is its relationship to glucose concentration. The rate at which Amadori products form is approximately proportional to the glucose concentration – double the glucose, roughly double the Amadori formation rate. But the conversion of Amadori products to AGEs involves oxidative steps whose rate depends on the square of the glucose concentration. This means that the relationship between blood sugar and AGE formation is not linear but exponential.

To make this concrete: a patient with average blood sugar corresponding to HbA1c 9% is not producing 1.5 times the AGE load of a patient at HbA1c 6%. They are producing approximately 2.25 times the AGE load – because 9/6 squared is 2.25. A patient at HbA1c 11% is producing nearly 3.4 times the AGE load of a patient at HbA1c 6%.

This square law has a direct implication for dietary management: small reductions in blood sugar produce disproportionately large reductions in AGE formation rate. Bringing HbA1c from 9% to 8% does not reduce your AGE production by 11%. It reduces it by approximately 20%. Bringing it from 9% to 7% reduces it by approximately 40%. Every percentage point of HbA1c reduction is more valuable than the percentage would suggest – because the AGE formation rate follows the square of the glucose concentration, not its linear value.

Dietary AGEs: The Pre-Formed Danger in Your Kitchen

There is a second source of AGEs in the body that is almost never discussed with patients: the AGEs that exist in food before it is eaten. When food is cooked using dry heat – grilling, frying, broiling, roasting – the same Maillard reaction that runs slowly at body temperature runs rapidly at cooking temperatures. The AGEs produced during cooking are partially absorbed through the gut wall and enter the circulation, adding to the total AGE burden the body is managing.

The difference between cooking methods is dramatic. A chicken breast that is grilled contains approximately 9,000 kilo-units of AGEs per 100 grams. The same chicken breast that is poached or steamed contains approximately 900 kilo-units — a tenfold difference. A piece of bacon fried until crispy contains roughly 90,000 kilo-units per 100 grams. A soft-boiled egg contains approximately 90 kilo-units. The cooking method is not a minor variable in AGE exposure — it is one of the most important dietary determinants of AGE intake.[4]

Dry high-heat cooking produces dramatically more advanced glycation end-products than moist low-heat methods

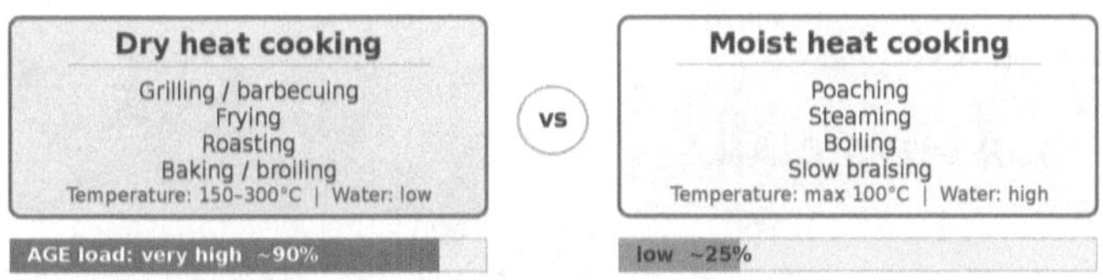

AGE content — chicken breast, different cooking methods

Method	Temp (°C)	AGE units (kU)	vs grilled
Grilled / broiled	200-260	~5,200 kU	—
Roasted	180-200	~4,300 kU	−17%
Pan fried	160-180	~2,400 kU	−54%
Boiled / poached	100	~1,000 kU	−81%
Steamed	100	~900 kU	−83%

The single most impactful cooking change for T2DM

Switching from grilling to poaching or steaming reduces dietary AGE intake by over 80% — a larger effect than most dietary supplements produce on AGE levels, at zero cost.

FIGURE 2. AGE formation by cooking method: grilling vs poaching — an eightfold difference in dietary AGE load.

Marinating food in acidic solutions before dry-heat cooking — lemon juice, vinegar, wine — reduces AGE formation during cooking by approximately 50%, because the acidic environment interferes with the Schiff base formation step. Acidic marinades do not eliminate the effect of dry heat, but they substantially reduce it.[5]

WHAT THIS MEANS FOR YOU

THE BOTTOM LINE

Your blood sugar is reacting with your proteins right now. The reaction is slow at body temperature, but it never stops, and its products are permanent. Every dietary choice you make either speeds that reaction or slows it. The most important thing you can learn from this chapter is that small improvements in blood sugar control produce disproportionately large reductions in the rate of this chemistry — because the reaction rate follows the square of the glucose concentration, not its linear value. Small changes, made consistently, matter more than the numbers suggest.

FOR YOUR PHYSICIAN

The Maillard reaction's kinetics in physiological conditions: Brownlee M, *Nature* 2001;414:813–820 remains the foundational mechanistic reference. The square-law dependence of AGE formation on glucose concentration is described in detail in Monnier VM et al., *Diabetes Care* 1999;22:B16–B23.

Dietary AGE content by food and cooking method: Uribarri J et al., *J Am Diet Assoc* 2010;110(6):911–916. The acidic marinade intervention: Uribarri J et al., Diabetes Care 2011;34:1314–1319.

CHAPTER 2

The Network and Its Amplifiers

Robert and James are both fifty-eight years old. Both were diagnosed with type 2 diabetes eight years ago. Both have maintained an average HbA1c of 8.2% throughout those eight years — not perfect, but consistent. Both are on the same medications. Both see the same type of physician. Both received the same dietary counseling at diagnosis.

Last month, Robert received the news that his kidney function has declined significantly. His urinary albumin-to-creatinine ratio, which was normal three years ago, is now 285 mg/g — well into the macroalbuminuria range. His nephrologist has told him that without significant changes, he is on a trajectory toward dialysis within ten years.

James, meanwhile, has been told that his kidneys are fine — but that his retinal examination shows moderate non-proliferative diabetic retinopathy. Micro-aneurysms and hard exudates are visible on fundoscopy. His ophthalmologist has recommended laser photocoagulation if the retinopathy progresses.

Robert's kidneys. James's eyes. Same blood sugar for the same number of years. Same treatment. Different organs affected first.

For decades, this kind of variation was explained as bad luck — individual susceptibility, genetic differences, random chance. That explanation was never fully satisfying, and in the past twenty years it has been replaced by something more precise: the concept of the hyperglycemic damage network. Understanding this network is the key to understanding not only why Robert's kidneys are failing while

James's eyes are deteriorating, but also why the dietary interventions described in Part II of this book are targeted at specific nodes of that network rather than just at blood sugar reduction in general.

THE SCIENCE BEHIND THIS

Seven Nodes, One Network

The advanced glycation end-products described in Chapter 1 are the entry point to a damage network with seven interconnected nodes. The glycation cascade itself is the first node – the chemistry described in Chapter 1, which generates the AGE products that initiate the cascade. Five additional pathway nodes amplify the damage in parallel, each one targeting different tissues through different mechanisms. A seventh node – the NF-κB inflammatory loop – receives signals from all five amplifying pathways and converges them into the tissue damage that produces clinical complications.

These seven nodes are not separate diseases. They are one disease expressed through interconnected pathways that reinforce and accelerate each other. Understanding the network structure is the most important conceptual shift in modern diabetes biology, and it explains something that a list of complications never could: why the damage is progressive, why it continues even when blood sugar is normalized, and why some interventions produce benefits that exceed what their glucose-lowering effect alone would predict.

The Seven Nodes at a Glance

The seven nodes of the damage network divide naturally into three functional groups: the entry node, where blood glucose first becomes chemistry; five amplifying nodes, where the chemistry spreads into specific cellular pathways; and the convergence node, where all five amplifying pathways feed into a self-sustaining inflammatory loop.

Node 1 – GCN: The Glycation Cascade

This is the entry node, described in detail in Chapter 1. Glucose bonds to proteins through the Maillard reaction, producing Schiff bases, then Amadori products, then Advanced Glycation End-Products. AGEs are essentially permanent. They accumulate in long-lived tissue proteins for years. They also bind to RAGE receptors, initiating the inflammatory signaling that feeds the convergence node. Methylglyoxal – a reactive carbonyl that reacts with proteins 20,000 times faster than glucose itself – is produced as a side product of accelerated glucose metabolism and contributes the most damaging AGEs in diabetic tissues.

Elevated blood glucose activates a self-amplifying network of seven molecular pathways.

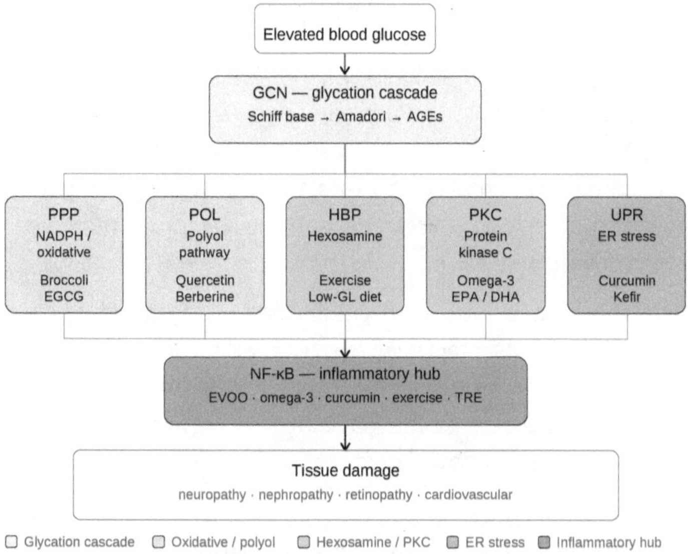

FIGURE 3. The seven-node T2DM damage network — glycation cascade and its six amplifying pathways.

Nodes 2 through 6 — The Five Amplifying Pathways

Chronic hyperglycemia activates five additional molecular pathways, each one targeting different tissues through different mechanisms. These pathways do not simply run in parallel — they amplify each other, share intermediates, and connect through the central mechanism of mitochondrial superoxide production that links them all. Chapter 3 describes each in detail and identifies the dietary intervention specific to each.

- **Node 2 — PPP:** The pentose phosphate pathway, whose impairment depletes the cell's antioxidant defenses.
- **Node 3 — POL:** The polyol pathway, which converts glucose to sorbitol in nerve and lens cells, producing osmotic damage.
- **Node 4 — HBP:** The hexosamine pathway, which makes insulin resistance progressively worse at the molecular level.
- **Node 5 — PKC:** Protein kinase C activation, which drives blood vessel damage in the retina and kidney.
- **Node 6 — UPR:** The endoplasmic reticulum stress response, which ultimately drives cell death and feeds back into inflammation.

Node 7 – NF-κB: The Inflammatory Convergence

All five amplifying pathways feed into the activation of NF-κB – Nuclear Factor kappa-light-chain-enhancer of activated B cells[6] – one of the most important transcription factors in human biology. When NF-κB is activated, it switches on the expression of over 150 inflammatory genes including TNF-alpha, IL-6, VCAM-1, ICAM-1, and – critically – RAGE itself. This last point is the reason the loop becomes self-amplifying: AGEs activate NF-κB through RAGE, and NF-κB makes more RAGE, which means the cell becomes more sensitive to AGEs, which drives more NF-κB, which makes more RAGE.

> Once this loop is sufficiently established – after years of elevated blood sugar – it can sustain itself even when blood sugar is normalized. The inflammation continues running on its own momentum, independent of the glucose that started it. This is one of the molecular mechanisms of metabolic memory, which we will explore fully in Chapter 4.

Two Mechanisms That Cross the Whole Network

Beyond the seven nodes, two molecular mechanisms operate across the entire network and deserve mention here because they explain how the nodes interconnect. The first is mitochondrial superoxide production. In 2001, the biochemist Michael Brownlee published a landmark paper in Nature showing that overloaded mitochondria in hyperglycemic cells produce excess superoxide, and that this superoxide is the central upstream mechanism that activates all five amplifying pathways simultaneously. When he added a mitochondrial antioxidant to cells grown in high glucose, all five pathways were simultaneously inhibited. The energy hijacker drives everything.[7]

The second is epigenetic reprogramming – the chemical marks on the proteins that package DNA, which translate the network's signaling into lasting changes in gene expression. Chapter 4 covers this mechanism in detail. Together with the NF-κB convergence node, the epigenetic mechanism explains why the network can sustain itself even after blood sugar is normalized.

Why Robert's Kidneys and James's Eyes

The network model explains the variation between Robert and James. Both have the same average blood sugar, but the distribution of node activation differs between them. Robert's network is dominant in the polyol (Node 3) and protein kinase C (Node 5) nodes – the pathways that most directly drive glomerular basement membrane thickening and mesangial expansion. James's network is dominant in the PKC node at the retinal level, where pericyte loss from PKC-beta activation produces the micro-aneurysms his ophthalmologist sees on fundoscopy.

These differences in network activation pattern reflect genetic variation in the enzymes of each pathway, differences in the local glucose environment in different tissues, and differences in the cross-pathway amplification dynamics. They are not random. They are the predictable output of a network whose specific activation pattern determines which organ is affected first.

WHAT THIS MEANS FOR YOU

THE BOTTOM LINE

The complications of diabetes are not separate bad outcomes that happen to affect different organs. They are the outputs of one interconnected molecular network that elevated blood sugar activates. The network has positive feedback loops – mechanisms by which each node amplifies the others – that can make it self-sustaining over time. Understanding the network changes the dietary question from 'what should I avoid?' to 'which nodes can I suppress?' Part II answers that question, node by node, food by food.

FOR YOUR PHYSICIAN

The unifying mechanism of hyperglycemic damage via mitochondrial superoxide: Brownlee M, *Nature* 2001;414:813–820. The seminal paper establishing the central role of mitochondrial ROS in activating all four classical biochemical pathways.

RAGE biology and the NF-κB amplification loop: Schmidt AM et al., *Circ Res* 1999;84:489–497. RAGE as a multiligand receptor: Bucciarelli LG et al., *Cell Mol Life Sci* 2002;59:1117–1128.

Methylglyoxal and glyoxalase I: Rabbani N, Thornalley PJ, *Antioxid Redox Signal* 2019;30:354–374.[8]

CHAPTER 3

Six More Reasons the Chemistry Is Running

A cardiologist once told me something that changed the way I explain diabetes to my patients. She said: "I can predict which of my heart failure patients have diabetes before I look at their chart. Not from their weight, not from their labs — from their echocardiogram. The heart failure pattern is different." She was describing diabetic cardiomyopathy: the stiffening of heart muscle from AGE cross-links in the myocardial collagen that produces a specific pattern of diastolic dysfunction visible on ultrasound. It is a complication that has nothing to do with blocked coronary arteries. It is the direct imprint of the Maillard reaction on cardiac tissue.

But she also made another observation: "The SGLT2 inhibitors do something to the diabetic heart that their blood-sugar-lowering effect alone doesn't explain. The cardiac benefit is too large, and it happens too quickly. Something else is going on."

She was right. Something else is going on — and it involves the six additional metabolic pathway disruptions that run in parallel with the glycation cascade described in Chapter 2. These six pathways help explain why SGLT2 inhibitors reduce heart failure hospitalizations by 35% in patients who barely needed them for glycemic control. They explain why green tea consumption is associated with lower rates of type 2 diabetes complications in epidemiological studies. They explain why certain dietary patterns produce metabolic benefits that cannot be attributed to caloric restriction alone.

This chapter introduces the six pathways. Part II will show you the foods and habits that intervene on each one.

THE SCIENCE BEHIND THIS

Pathway 1 — The Energy Factory Running Too Hot: TCA Cycle Disruption

The tricarboxylic acid cycle — also called the Krebs cycle or TCA cycle — is the central metabolic hub of every cell. It takes the two-carbon acetyl-CoA produced from glucose, fatty acids, and amino acids and extracts energy from it through eight enzymatic steps, producing the NADH and FADH2 that power the electron transport chain. Under normal conditions, the TCA cycle turns at a rate matched to the cell's energy demands. Under chronic hyperglycemia, it is flooded with substrate — more acetyl-CoA than the enzymes can process efficiently.

The overloaded TCA cycle accumulates its intermediates. The most consequential of these is succinate. Under normal conditions, succinate is rapidly oxidized to fumarate. When it accumulates, it inhibits the enzymes that tag a protein called HIF-1alpha for destruction. HIF-1alpha is the cell's hypoxia sensor — the protein that gets switched on when oxygen is scarce and drives the expression of VEGF, anaerobic metabolism genes, and inflammatory macrophage activation. When succinate accumulates in a well-oxygenated diabetic cell, HIF-1alpha is stabilized as if the cell were oxygen-deprived. The cell responds to a false hypoxia signal, producing VEGF in the retina and activating inflammatory macrophages throughout the body.[9]

This is the mechanistic explanation for a dietary intervention described in Part IV: why time-restricted eating and fasting reduce TCA cycle substrate overload and improve mitochondrial efficiency. And it is part of the explanation for why SGLT2 inhibitors, which reduce the glucose available to the TCA cycle and stimulate ketone body production that activates a mitochondrial biogenesis pathway called PGC-1alpha, produce cardiovascular benefits beyond their glucose-lowering effect.

Pathway 2 — The Antioxidant Depletion: Pentose Phosphate Pathway Impairment

The pentose phosphate pathway (PPP) branches off from the main glucose metabolism pathway at glucose-6-phosphate. Its most important function is to produce NADPH — the molecule that powers the entire antioxidant defense system of the cell. NADPH is required by glutathione reductase, which regenerates the reduced glutathione that neutralizes reactive oxygen species. NADPH is required by the enzyme that produces nitric oxide in endothelial cells. NADPH is required by catalase, which breaks down hydrogen peroxide. Without adequate NADPH, the cell's ability to neutralize oxidative stress collapses.

In the hyperglycemic environment, PPP flux is impaired by the same mechanism that activates all four classical damage pathways: inhibition of the glycolytic enzyme GAPDH by the superoxide produced in Node 2. When GAPDH is inhibited, the upstream glycolytic intermediates accumulate and are redirected into the PPP at abnormal rates, disrupting its normal function and ultimately depleting NADPH.

The food-based intervention for this pathway — sulforaphane from broccoli sprouts, riboflavin from dairy and leafy greens, benfotiamine from thiamine-rich foods — is described in Chapter 7. The core principle: the PPP can be partly rehabilitated by providing the cofactors it needs and activating the transcription factor Nrf2, which upregulates the entire antioxidant gene program.

Pathway 3 — The Sorbitol Trap: The Polyol Pathway

Normally, glucose is metabolized almost entirely through glycolysis and the TCA cycle. A minor side pathway exists — the polyol pathway — that converts glucose to sorbitol through an enzyme called aldose reductase, then converts sorbitol to fructose through another enzyme called sorbitol dehydrogenase. Under normal blood sugar conditions, this pathway handles less than 3% of glucose metabolism, because aldose reductase has low affinity for glucose at physiological concentrations.

In hyperglycemia, intracellular glucose concentrations rise in tissues where glucose entry does not depend on insulin — the lens of the eye, the peripheral nerves, the kidney, the retina. In these tissues, aldose reductase becomes active and diverts significant glucose flux into the polyol pathway. The consequences are multiple: sorbitol accumulates because it cannot cross cell membranes easily, creating osmotic stress that damages cell structure. The NADPH consumed by aldose reductase reduces the cell's antioxidant capacity (amplifying Pathway 2). The NAD+ consumed by sorbitol dehydrogenase depletes a cofactor needed by SIRT1, the enzyme that maintains the protective epigenetic marks described in the next chapter.

The lens is the most directly affected tissue: sorbitol accumulation in the lens cells disrupts the crystallin proteins that maintain lens transparency, producing the characteristic nuclear cataract of diabetes. In peripheral nerves, sorbitol accumulation from Schwann cell polyol pathway activity contributes to the osmotic damage underlying diabetic neuropathy. Quercetin, the flavonoid abundant in onions, capers, and apples, is one of the most potent naturally occurring aldose reductase inhibitors known — a dietary intervention directly targeted at this pathway. We will cover it in Chapter 8.

Pathway 4 — The Insulin Resistance Amplifier: The Hexosamine Pathway

Approximately 2 to 3% of normal glucose flux is diverted into the hexosamine biosynthetic pathway, producing a molecule called UDP-GlcNAc. This molecule is the substrate for an enzyme called O-GlcNAc transferase (OGT), which attaches GlcNAc groups to serine and threonine residues on proteins — the same amino acid residues that protein kinases attach phosphate groups to in order to activate or inhibit protein function.

This O-GlcNAc modification competes with phosphorylation. When the hexosamine pathway is overactive in hyperglycemia, O-GlcNAc modification displaces the activating phosphorylation on key insulin signaling proteins — specifically on insulin receptor substrate-1 (IRS-1) and on the kinase Akt. The result is progressive insulin resistance: the more glucose that flows through the hexosamine pathway, the more insulin signaling is impaired, the less glucose the cell takes up, the higher blood sugar stays. This is a vicious cycle that makes insulin resistance self-amplifying at the molecular level.

Dietary carbohydrate restriction — reducing the amount of glucose flowing through glycolysis — directly reduces hexosamine pathway flux. Berberine, the plant alkaloid discussed in Chapter 9, activates AMPK, which reduces hexosamine pathway activity by diverting glucose flux away from the pathway's substrate. This is one of the reasons berberine's insulin-sensitizing effect parallels that of metformin.

Pathway 5 — The Blood Vessel Damage Driver: Protein Kinase C

Protein kinase C (PKC) is a family of enzymes activated by diacylglycerol (DAG), a lipid second messenger. Under hyperglycemic conditions, DAG accumulates in cells through two mechanisms: increased synthesis from glycolytic intermediates, and impaired degradation by DAG kinase (which is inhibited by oxidative stress from Pathway 2). The excess DAG.activates PKC, particularly the beta and delta isoforms.

PKC-beta activation in retinal cells drives VEGF overexpression — the signal that stimulates the abnormal blood vessel growth of proliferative diabetic retinopathy. PKC-beta activation in glomerular mesangial cells drives TGF-beta production, fibronectin synthesis, and collagen IV deposition that thicken the glomerular basement membrane and progressively impair kidney filtration. PKC activation in endothelial cells impairs eNOS activation, reducing nitric oxide production and contributing to the endothelial dysfunction that underlies macrovascular disease.[10]

The omega-3 fatty acids EPA and DHA, found in fatty fish and fish oil, incorporate into cell membranes and displace the arachidonic acid that is a precursor to DAG, directly reducing PKC activation. This mechanism is one of the explanations for omega-3s' specific benefits for retinopathy and nephropathy in diabetic patients — effects that go beyond their well-documented anti-inflammatory properties.

Pathway 6 — The Protein Factory in Crisis: Endoplasmic Reticulum Stress

The endoplasmic reticulum (ER) is the cell's protein synthesis and quality-control factory. Every protein destined for secretion or insertion into the cell membrane passes through the ER, where it is folded into its correct three-dimensional shape by a team of chaperone proteins. When too many misfolded or abnormal proteins accumulate in the ER — as happens when AGE-modified proteins are produced faster than the folding machinery can handle them — the ER activates a stress response called the Unfolded Protein Response (UPR).

The UPR has three branches. When mild and transient, it is protective: it upregulates chaperone production, reduces protein synthesis to give the factory time to catch up, and activates pathways that clear misfolded proteins. When chronic and severe — as it becomes in long-standing diabetes — the UPR transitions from protective to destructive. It activates a protein called CHOP that drives cell apoptosis, contributing to the beta-cell loss that accelerates insulin deficiency over time. It activates JNK signaling, which directly impairs IRS-1 function and worsens insulin resistance through the same serine phosphorylation site targeted by the hexosamine pathway. And it activates NF-κB through IRE1-alpha signaling, feeding back into the inflammatory amplification loop of Node 1.[11]

The dietary intervention for ER stress is among the most fascinating in this book: EGCG from green tea inhibits IRE1-alpha, reducing UPR activation. Tauroursodeoxycholic acid (TUDCA), a bile acid derivative found in small amounts in some fermented foods and available as a supplement, is one of the most potent chemical chaperones known and directly reduces the ER's protein-folding burden. We cover both in Chapter 11.

The Complete Picture

The five amplifying pathways described in this chapter — together with the glycation cascade of Chapter 1 and the NF-κB inflammatory convergence introduced in Chapter 2 — constitute the seven-node hyperglycemic damage network: the complete molecular architecture of diabetic tissue damage. Each node is a target. Each target has dietary interventions. Part II of this book addresses them systematically, with specific food choices, preparation methods, and evidence-based supplements for each.

WHAT THIS MEANS FOR YOU

THE BOTTOM LINE

Six additional molecular pathways run in parallel with the glycation cascade, each one amplifying the others and each one addressable through specific dietary choices. The TCA cycle overload produces false hypoxia signals. The pentose phosphate pathway impairment depletes your antioxidant defenses. The polyol pathway traps nerve and lens cells in a sorbitol accumulation. The hexosamine pathway makes your insulin resistance progressively worse. The PKC pathway drives blood vessel damage in the retina and kidney. ER stress drives cell death and feeds back into inflammation. Part II shows you what to eat to intervene on each one.

FOR YOUR PHYSICIAN

The six classical biochemical pathways of hyperglycemic damage unified by mitochondrial superoxide: Brownlee M, *Nature* 2001;414:813–820.

TCA cycle disruption and succinate as a HIF-1alpha stabilizer in diabetes: Mills EL et al., *Nat Immunol* 2017;18:488–498.

Polyol pathway and diabetic complications: Lorenzi M, *Exp Diabetes Res* 2007;2007:61038. Aldose reductase inhibition by quercetin: literature reviewed in Costantino L et al., *J Med Chem 1999;42:1881–1893.*

Hexosamine pathway and O-GlcNAc interference with insulin signaling: Hart GW et al., Annu Rev Biochem 2011;80:825–858.

PKC-beta and diabetic retinopathy: Geraldes P, King GL, *Circ Res* 2010;106:1319–1331.

ER stress in T2DM: Hotamisligil GS, *Cell* 2010;140:900–917.

CHAPTER 4

The Memory Your Body Keeps

In 1993, a clinical trial ended. The Diabetes Control and Complications Trial — the DCCT — had spent nearly a decade following 1,441 patients with type 1 diabetes, randomized to either intensive glycemic control (target HbA1c around 7%) or conventional control (target HbA1c around 9%). The intensive group had dramatically lower rates of retinopathy, nephropathy, and neuropathy. The result was not surprising — everyone expected intensive control to be better. What happened next was surprising.[12]

When the trial ended, both groups were counseled to adopt intensive glycemic control. Within a few years, the HbA1c levels of the two groups had converged. There was no longer a meaningful difference in blood sugar between patients who had been in the intensive group and those who had been in the conventional group.

Yet when the researchers continued following these patients for another ten years, something remarkable emerged. The patients who had been in the intensive group — the ones who had maintained better blood sugar during the trial — continued to have lower rates of cardiovascular events, nephropathy, and neuropathy. Not because their blood sugar was currently better — it was now the same. But because their history of blood sugar had been better. The benefit of those years of good control persisted for a decade after the advantage had been erased.[13]

The researchers called this phenomenon metabolic memory. It has since been replicated in the UKPDS 80 legacy study for type 2 diabetes, where the group originally randomized to intensive therapy maintained a cardiovascular mortality benefit for ten years after the trial, even after HbA1c levels equalized between groups.[14]

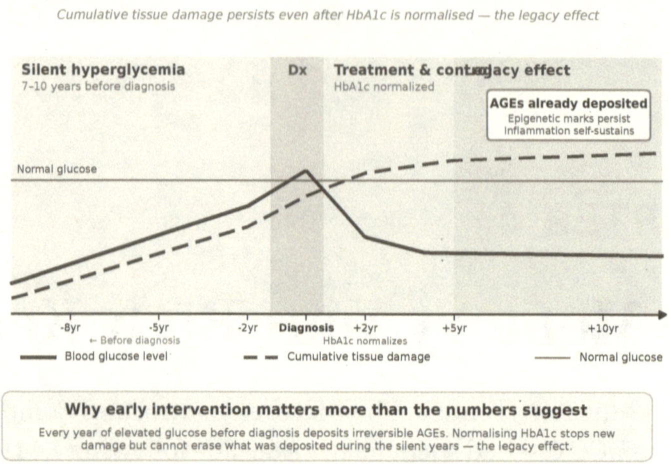

FIGURE 4. The legacy effect: cumulative tissue damage persists even after HbA1c is normalised.

For years, metabolic memory was acknowledged but unexplained. It was a clinical observation without a molecular mechanism — a fact that demanded interpretation. In 2008, a paper in the Journal of Experimental Medicine by El-Osta and colleagues provided the first molecular explanation, and it involved a biological process that most patients with T2DM have never heard of: epigenetics.[15]

THE SCIENCE BEHIND THIS

What Epigenetics Means: The User's Guide to Your DNA Packaging

Your DNA contains approximately 3 billion base pairs encoding roughly 20,000 genes. If it were stretched out end to end, the DNA from a single cell would extend about two meters. It fits inside a cell nucleus that is approximately 6 micrometers in diameter – roughly 1/17th the thickness of a human hair – because it is wound tightly around protein spools called histones, coiled and compacted into a structure called chromatin.

The packaging is not merely a space-saving arrangement. It is a regulatory system. Genes that are tightly wrapped around histones cannot be read by the cell's transcription machinery – they are effectively switched off. Genes that are loosely arranged, with the DNA accessible to transcription factors, can be read and expressed. The state of DNA packaging – how tightly or loosely each gene is wound around its histones – is the primary mechanism by which cells control which of their 20,000 genes are active at any given moment.

The marks that determine packaging state are chemical modifications to the histone proteins themselves: acetyl groups, methyl groups, phosphate groups, and others can be attached to or removed from specific amino acid positions on the histones. These marks are written by specialized enzymes (histone acetyltransferases, histone methyltransferases), erased by other enzymes (deacetylases, demethylases), and read by yet another set of proteins that determine whether a gene is transcribed. Different combinations of marks at different positions produce different states of gene activation — a histone code that regulates gene expression with extraordinary specificity.

The critical feature of this histone code for our purposes is that it is heritable. When a cell divides, the histone marks on the parent cell's chromatin are largely reproduced on the daughter cells' chromatin. The regulatory state — which genes are active, which are suppressed — is passed from parent cell to daughter cell through the marks on the histones, not through changes in the DNA sequence itself. This is the essence of epigenetics: gene regulation through mechanisms other than DNA sequence, capable of persisting across cell divisions.

How Elevated Blood Sugar Writes Into Chromatin

The El-Osta group's 2008 paper demonstrated the specific molecular sequence through which transient high glucose exposure — even exposure lasting only a few days — produces lasting epigenetic changes at inflammatory gene promoters in vascular endothelial cells.

The sequence begins with AGE-RAGE signaling, which we met in Chapter 2. RAGE activation by AGEs causes the NF-κB subunit p65 to translocate into the cell nucleus. Once in the nucleus, p65 does not merely activate NF-κB target genes in the conventional sense — it also recruits a histone methyltransferase enzyme called Set7/9 to the promoters of those target genes. Set7/9 deposits the histone mark H3K4me1 — a monomethylation of lysine 4 on histone H3 — at those promoters. H3K4me1 is an active chromatin mark: it loosens the DNA from the histone, making the gene accessible to the transcription machinery.

At the same time, NF-κB activation drives the enzyme PARP-1 to deplete the cell's supply of NAD+ — the cofactor that a deacetylase enzyme called SIRT1 requires to do its job. SIRT1 is the enzyme responsible for maintaining the repressive chromatin state at inflammatory gene promoters: it removes acetyl groups from histones and enables the addition of repressive methyl marks. When SIRT1 loses its NAD+ supply, it cannot maintain the repressive marks, and the activating marks written by Set7/9 go unopposed.

The result: inflammatory gene promoters — including the promoters of NF-κB target genes, VCAM-1, MCP-1, and RAGE itself — transition from a repressed state to an activated state. This transition is stable. When blood sugar is normalized, Set7/9 stops depositing new H3K4me1 marks at these promoters, but the marks that are already there are not immediately removed. They persist through multiple cell divisions. The cell's inflammatory program remains switched on at a level determined by the history of blood sugar exposure, not the current blood sugar.

This is the molecular mechanism of metabolic memory. The years of elevated blood sugar in the DCCT conventional control group had written activating marks into the chromatin at inflammatory promoters in vascular endothelial cells, macrophages, and other cell types throughout the vasculature. When blood sugar was normalized at the trial's end, the glucose was gone but the marks remained — and they continued to drive the inflammatory and fibrotic processes that produce cardiovascular events, nephropathy, and retinopathy.

SIRT1: The Enzyme at the Center

SIRT1 — Sirtuin 1 — occupies a central position in this story that extends far beyond its role in histone deacetylation. SIRT1 is activated by caloric restriction and by the chemical signal of an energy-depleted state: the ratio of NAD+ to NADH. When cells are well-fed, NAD+ is converted to NADH during metabolism, and SIRT1 activity declines. When cells are fasted or calorically restricted, NAD+ rises relative to NADH, and SIRT1 becomes active.[16]

Active SIRT1 does many things simultaneously: it deacetylates the inflammatory gene promoters described above, maintaining their repressive state. It activates PGC-1alpha, driving mitochondrial biogenesis and improving the cell's ability to handle metabolic substrate without producing oxidative stress. It activates FOXO transcription factors that drive antioxidant gene expression. And it deacetylates and activates LKB1, which activates AMPK — the master metabolic sensor.

The fasting state activates SIRT1. Intermittent fasting activates SIRT1. Several polyphenols activate SIRT1 directly or indirectly. Resveratrol, the stilbene from red grapes and blueberries, was initially identified as a SIRT1 activator in the early 2000s and sparked an enormous research interest in SIRT1's role in metabolism, aging, and disease. The complete story of dietary

SIRT1 activation is told in Part IV and Part V. But the concept is important enough to introduce here: when you activate SIRT1 through fasting or through specific plant compounds, you are not doing something vaguely 'healthy.' You are activating the epigenetic eraser that opposes the inflammatory marks written by years of elevated blood sugar.

DNA Methylation: The Deeper Layer

Histone modification is not the only epigenetic mechanism altered by chronic hyperglycemia. DNA itself can be chemically modified by the addition of methyl groups directly to cytosine bases in the DNA sequence – particularly at CpG dinucleotides in gene promoter regions. DNA methylation at a gene promoter generally silences that gene. Demethylation generally activates it.

In the context of the damage network, two DNA methylation changes are particularly consequential. First, the promoter of the SIRT1 gene itself undergoes progressive methylation in hyperglycemic environments, reducing SIRT1 expression at the transcriptional level – adding a second mechanism of SIRT1 suppression on top of the NAD+ depletion mechanism described above. Second, the promoters of certain antioxidant defense genes undergo methylation-driven silencing in diabetic vasculature, reducing the cell's ability to respond to oxidative stress.[17]

DNA methylation changes are more stable than histone modifications – they are replicated with high fidelity during cell division and are not reversed by the enzymes that remove histone marks. This makes DNA methylation-based epigenetic changes the most persistent form of metabolic memory, and it explains why some of the legacy effects of poor glycemic control may persist for the lifetime of the affected cell population.

What This Means for the Timing of Intervention

The epigenetic mechanism of metabolic memory has one clinical implication that overrides all others: the value of early intervention is not proportional to the HbA1c difference it produces. It is proportional to the amount of epigenetic modification it prevents.

A patient who achieves HbA1c 7% in their first year of diagnosis has prevented the accumulation of inflammatory histone marks at a time when they are not yet established. A patient who achieves the same HbA1c 7% after ten years of HbA1c 9% has reduced the ongoing production of those marks – a genuine and important benefit – but cannot fully erase the marks already written.

The chromatin state of their vascular endothelium carries the record of those ten years, and that record continues to drive inflammatory gene expression.

This is why Chapter 1's conclusion – that the square law of AGE formation makes early intervention disproportionately valuable – applies even more strongly to the epigenetic dimension of the disease. Early control does not merely slow AGE accumulation faster. It prevents the writing of epigenetic marks that, once written, have no pharmacological eraser currently available.

WHAT THIS MEANS FOR YOU

THE BOTTOM LINE

Your cells remember your blood sugar history. The memory is written in the chemical marks on the proteins that package your DNA, and it persists for years after blood sugar is normalized. This is metabolic memory – and it is the molecular explanation for why patients who had good blood sugar control early in their diabetes had better cardiovascular outcomes a decade later, even after their blood sugar advantage had been erased. The most powerful response to this fact is not despair but urgency: the epigenetic record is still being written right now, and the choices you make today determine what is written. SIRT1 – activated by fasting and by specific plant compounds – is the cell's own mechanism for opposing the inflammatory record. Part IV and Part V show you how to activate it.

FOR YOUR PHYSICIAN

The metabolic memory phenomenon in DCCT/EDIC: Nathan DM et al., *N Engl J Med* 2005;353:2643–2653. The molecular mechanism via histone methylation: El-Osta A et al., *J Exp Med* 2008;205:2409–2417. Confirmation of H3K4me1 deposition at NF-κB promoters: Brasacchio D et al., *Diabetes* 2009;58:1229–1236.[18]

SIRT1 in metabolic regulation and epigenetic maintenance: Canto C, Auwerx J, *Cell Metab* 2009;11:449–460.

DNA methylation changes at the SIRT1 promoter in diabetic vascular tissue: Villeneuve LM et al., *Diabetes* 2010;59:1783–1791.

UKPDS 80 legacy effects: Holman RR et al., *N Engl J Med* 2008;359:1577–1589.

Closing Reflection on Part I

Part I has covered four chapters and a substantial amount of biology. If it has done its job, you now understand something that no dietary guideline will ever tell you: the mechanism by which food choices affect your disease.

> You know that glucose reacts with your proteins through a chemical pathway that produces irreversible products at a rate proportional to the square of your blood sugar concentration — which means that small improvements in control produce disproportionately large benefits.
>
> You know that this glycation reaction is the entry point to a network of seven interconnected nodes — five amplifying pathways that each target different tissues, plus the inflammatory convergence node that allows the damage to sustain itself even when blood sugar is normalized.
>
> You know that the network can eventually sustain itself without elevated glucose, through the inflammatory amplification loop, through ER stress, through depleted SIRT1 — and that this self-sustaining capacity is the molecular mechanism of metabolic memory.
>
> And you know that SIRT1 — activated by fasting and by specific plant compounds — is your cells' own mechanism for opposing the inflammatory epigenetic record that elevated blood sugar writes.

Part II now shows you, node by node, which foods contain the molecular signals that suppress each pathway. The science is established. The foods are real. The changes are within your reach.

Part II

What Food Does to the Network

Every food you eat sends signals to the same molecular networkthat elevated blood sugar is damaging.Some foods amplify the damage. Some suppress it.Most people have never been told which is which.

Part I gave you the network. It described the seven molecular nodes through which elevated blood sugar damages tissue — the glycation cascade as the entry node, five amplifying pathways that target different tissues through different mechanisms, and the NF-kB inflammatory convergence node where the damage becomes self-sustaining. It explained why the damage is progressive, why it has memory, and why early intervention matters more than the numbers suggest.

Part II puts food against that map, node by node. Each chapter addresses one or two network nodes and identifies the specific foods, preparation methods, and evidence-based supplements that suppress that node's activity. The science is drawn from peer-reviewed clinical and laboratory research. The practical recommendations are derived directly from the mechanisms described — not from population studies of vague dietary patterns, but from the specific molecular pharmacology of specific compounds in specific foods.

A note on how to read Part II: you do not need to implement everything at once. Read the chapters in order. After each one, identify the one or two changes you will actually make. A person who makes three changes consistently for a year does more biological good than a person who attempts everything and sustains nothing. The network does not need to be suppressed all at once — it needs to be suppressed consistently.

CHAPTER 5

The Glycemic Hierarchy

Not All Carbohydrates Are the Same

David is a sixty-one-year-old retired teacher with type 2 diabetes diagnosed four years ago. He has been conscientious about his diet. He reads labels. He avoids candy and soda. He switched from regular bread to whole wheat bread three years ago, from white rice to brown rice two years ago, and from fruit juice to whole fruit one year ago. His HbA1c has improved modestly — from 8.4% at diagnosis to 7.8% now — but his physician has told him that further improvement is needed.

"I don't eat sugar," David says at his appointments. "I don't understand why my numbers aren't better."

The answer involves a distinction that most dietary counseling for diabetes fails to make clearly enough: the difference between glycemic index and glycemic load, and why the second one is the number that actually determines what happens to your blood sugar after a meal. David's brown rice is healthier than white rice in several ways — it contains more fiber, more magnesium, more B vitamins. But in terms of blood sugar impact, it produces a glucose spike that is only modestly smaller than white rice, because a standard serving of brown rice contains nearly the same amount of available carbohydrate.

Understanding the glycemic hierarchy does not require eliminating carbohydrates from your diet. It requires choosing them differently — and understanding the biology of why different carbohydrates produce such different responses in your body.

THE SCIENCE BEHIND THIS

Glycemic Index: The Speed of Sugar Entry

The glycemic index (GI) was developed by David Jenkins and colleagues at the University of Toronto in 1981. It measures how rapidly the carbohydrates in a given food raise blood glucose compared to a reference standard — either pure glucose (GI = 100) or white bread (GI = 100 in some scales). A food with a GI of 70 raises blood glucose approximately 70% as fast as pure glucose.[19]

The GI reflects the rate of carbohydrate digestion and absorption. Foods with high GI contain carbohydrates that are rapidly broken down by digestive enzymes — refined starches, sugars, and overcooked grains that have lost their structural integrity. Foods with low GI contain carbohydrates whose digestion is slowed by intact cell walls, resistant starch, fiber, fat, or protein content.

Several factors determine a food's GI. The type of starch matters: amylopectin, the branched form of starch, is more rapidly digestible than amylose, the linear form. Cooking matters: heat disrupts the crystalline structure of starch granules, making them more accessible to digestive enzymes — which is why freshly cooked rice and potatoes have higher GI than cooled and reheated versions of the same food. Processing matters: extruded breakfast cereals have high GI because the extrusion process extensively disrupts starch structure. Particle size matters: stone-ground whole wheat bread has a lower GI than finely milled whole wheat bread made with the same grain, because larger particles are digested more slowly.

Glycemic Load: The Amount of Blood Sugar Impact

Glycemic load (GL) extends the GI concept by incorporating the amount of carbohydrate in a realistic serving. It is calculated as: GL = GI × grams of available carbohydrate per serving ÷ 100.

This distinction matters enormously in practice. Watermelon has a high GI of approximately 72 — it is rapidly absorbed. But a standard serving of watermelon (about 120 grams) contains only about 6 grams of available carbohydrate, giving it a GL of only 4 — among the lowest of any food. Carrots present a similar situation: raw carrots have a GI of about 35, but a serving contains so little carbohydrate that their GL is negligible. By contrast, cooked parsnips have a similar GI to carrots but contain more carbohydrate per serving, producing a higher GL.

The most practically important GL comparison is between refined grains and whole grains. White rice has a GI of approximately 73 and a GL per standard serving (150g cooked) of approximately 43. Brown rice has a GI of approximately 66 and a GL per the same serving of approximately 38. The difference in blood sugar impact is real but modest — about 11%. This is why switching from white to brown rice is beneficial but not transformative for blood sugar management. The more impactful change is to reduce portion size of all rice, or to substitute rice with legumes (GL of cooked lentils per serving: approximately 7) or barley (GL approximately 11).[20]

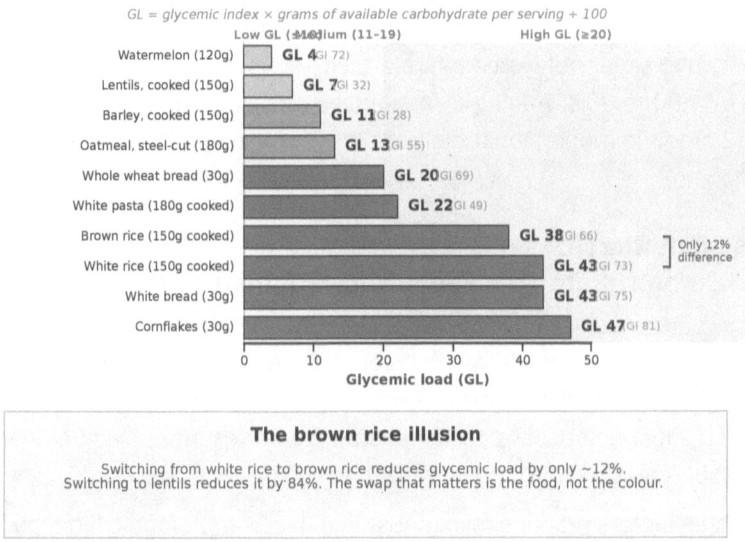

FIGURE 5. Glycemic load comparison: the same food choice produces very different blood glucose impacts.

The Fiber Modifier

Dietary fiber is not a single substance but a family of indigestible plant carbohydrates with diverse chemical structures and diverse metabolic effects. For blood sugar management, soluble fiber — the type that dissolves in water to form a viscous gel — is the most important. Beta-glucan from oats and barley, pectin from fruits, psyllium from plantain seeds, and the mucilage in okra and flaxseed are all soluble fibers that form gels in the small intestine.

These gels slow the movement of food through the gut and create a physical barrier between digestive enzymes and their starch substrates, reducing the rate of glucose absorption. They also trap bile acids, reducing cholesterol reabsorption and lowering LDL. And they ferment in the large intestine to produce short-chain fatty acids – butyrate, propionate, and acetate – that have direct anti-inflammatory effects and stimulate GLP-1 secretion from gut enteroendocrine cells.

The practical implication: adding a soluble fiber source to any carbohydrate-containing meal reduces that meal's glycemic impact. A bowl of oatmeal has a lower GL than the same calories of cornflakes not only because oats have lower GI but because beta-glucan slows the absorption of the oat starch. Adding psyllium to a glass of water before a meal reduces the subsequent glucose spike by 20 to 30%. Adding chia seeds – rich in soluble fiber – to yogurt or a smoothie moderates the glycemic response of everything consumed with them.[21]

Resistant Starch: The Carbohydrate That Feeds Your Gut Instead of Your Blood

Not all starch is digested in the small intestine. Resistant starch – starch that resists digestion by amylase and reaches the colon intact – is fermented by gut bacteria to produce short-chain fatty acids, just as soluble fiber is. From a blood sugar perspective, resistant starch behaves more like fiber than like digestible carbohydrate.

Three factors produce resistant starch in common foods. First, physical entrapment: intact cell walls in legumes, seeds, and coarsely ground grains prevent digestive enzymes from accessing the starch granules inside – which is why whole lentils have a dramatically lower glycemic impact than lentil flour, even though both contain the same total starch. Second, raw starch granule structure: raw potato and raw banana contain highly organized crystalline starch that resists enzymatic attack. Cooking disrupts this crystalline structure, increasing digestibility. Third – and most practically relevant for cooked foods – retrogradation: when cooked starch cools, some of the starch molecules reassemble into a more crystalline, enzyme-resistant form. Cooled and reheated rice, pasta, and potatoes contain more resistant starch than freshly cooked equivalents. This is not a trivial effect: cooling cooked rice for 12 hours reduces its digestible starch content by approximately 50%.[22]

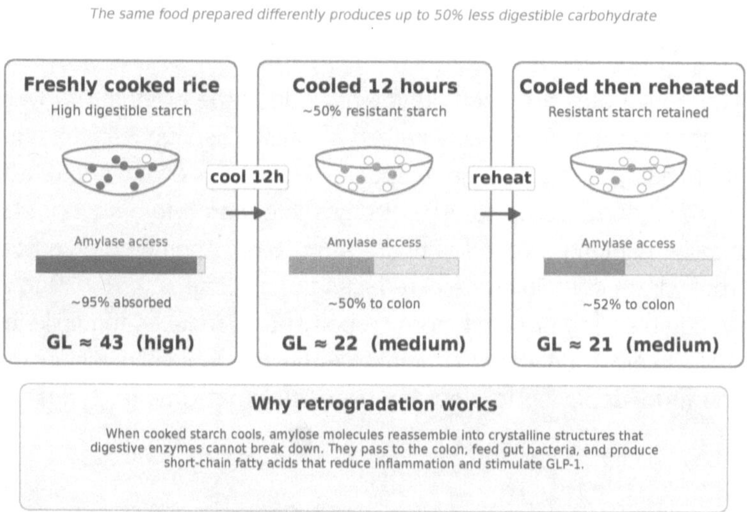

FIGURE 6. Resistant starch retrogradation: how cooling and reheating the same food transforms its glycemic impact.

The Cooking Method and AGE Intersection

Chapter 1 established that dry-heat cooking methods produce dramatically more dietary AGEs than moist-heat methods for animal proteins. For carbohydrate-containing foods, the same principle applies but through a different mechanism: the Maillard reaction between reducing sugars and amino acids at high temperatures produces not only browning and flavor compounds but also acrylamide — a potentially carcinogenic compound formed when asparagine (an amino acid in starchy foods) reacts with glucose at temperatures above 120°C. Roasted potatoes, toasted bread, and breakfast cereals processed at high temperatures all contain acrylamide in amounts that correlate with their degree of browning. Boiling, steaming, and microwaving produce minimal acrylamide because water limits the temperature to 100°C.

WHAT THIS MEANS FOR YOU

THE BOTTOM LINE

Not all carbohydrates are equal. Glycemic load – the product of glycemic index and the amount of carbohydrate in a realistic serving – is the number that determines your blood sugar response to a meal. Cooling and reheating cooked grains converts up to 50% of digestible starch to resistant starch, dramatically reducing glycemic impact at no cost. Adding soluble fiber to any carbohydrate-containing meal reduces the glucose spike by 20 to 30%. Eating vegetables and protein before carbohydrates reduces the spike by 30 to 40%. These are not dietary restrictions – they are tactical decisions about the same food, deployed to slow the chemistry that Chapter 1 described.

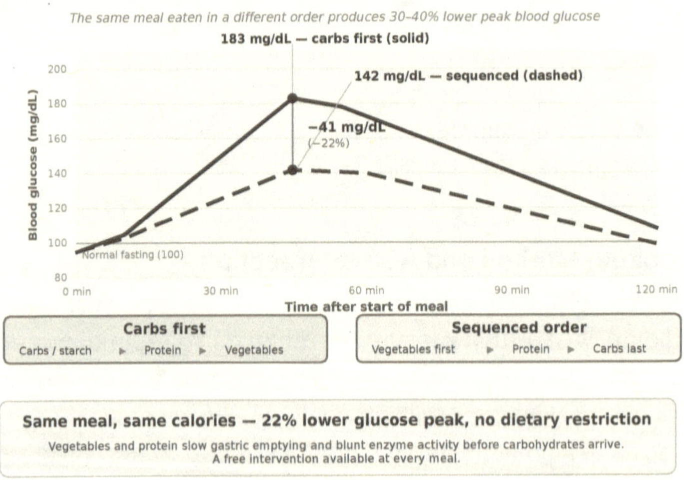

FIGURE 7. Food sequence and blood glucose: eating order reduces the glucose peak by 22% with no change in food.

FOR YOUR PHYSICIAN

Glycemic index methodology: Jenkins DJ et al., *Am J Clin Nutr* 1981;34:362–366. Comprehensive GI/GL tables: Atkinson FS et al., *Diabetes Care* 2008;31:2281–2283.

Resistant starch and postprandial glycemia: Birt DF et al., *Adv Nutr* 2013;4:587–601. Cooling rice reduces digestible starch content: Bodinham CL et al., *Br J Nutr* 2010;103:1213–1216.

Food sequence and postprandial glycemia: Shukla AP et al., *Diabetes Care* 2015;38:e98–e99. Replicated in: Nishino K et al., *J Clin Biochem Nutr* 2018;62:59–63.

Beta-glucan and glucose response: Tosh SM, *Food Hydrocoll* 2013;30:295–314.

CHAPTER 6

Fighting the Inflammatory Loop

Foods That Calm NF-κB

Patricia is sixty-seven years old and has had type 2 diabetes for twelve years. She also has osteoarthritis in her knees, and her rheumatologist has her on a low-dose NSAID. At her diabetes appointment, her physician notices that her inflammatory markers — hs-CRP and ferritin — are consistently elevated, suggesting that the inflammatory amplification loop described in Chapter 2 is running at a high level. Her HbA1c is 8.1%.

"I eat pretty well," she says. "Mostly Mediterranean." She means she uses olive oil and eats fish twice a week. She has the right idea — but she is applying it partially. The Mediterranean pattern's anti-inflammatory effect comes not from any single food but from the combination of several specific compounds, each one targeting the NF-κB inflammatory amplification loop described in Chapter 2 through a different molecular mechanism.

This chapter covers those compounds: the oleocanthal in high-quality extra virgin olive oil, the omega-3 fatty acids in fatty fish, and the curcumin in turmeric. Each one has been studied in isolation; together, they represent the most evidence-based dietary anti-inflammatory strategy available for T2DM patients.

THE SCIENCE BEHIND THIS

Oleocanthal: The Ibuprofen in Your Olive Oil

In 2005, Gary Beauchamp and colleagues at the Monell Chemical Senses Center published a paper in Nature that changed the way food scientists think about extra virgin olive oil. Beauchamp had noticed that freshly pressed extra virgin olive oil produced a distinct throat irritation – a burning sensation at the back of the throat – that resembled the throat sensation produced by ibuprofen taken as a liquid. On investigation, he identified the compound responsible: a phenolic aldehyde he named oleocanthal.[23, 24]

Oleocanthal inhibits both COX-1 and COX-2 – the same cyclooxygenase enzymes that ibuprofen inhibits – through the same mechanism, competitive inhibition. A 50-gram serving of extra virgin olive oil delivers approximately 9 milligrams of oleocanthal, which corresponds to roughly 10% of the ibuprofen dose in a standard 200mg tablet. This is not a trivial pharmacological effect: consumed at every meal over a lifetime, this daily low-dose COX inhibition produces a sustained anti-inflammatory signal that partially suppresses the prostaglandin and thromboxane production that amplifies the NF-κB loop.

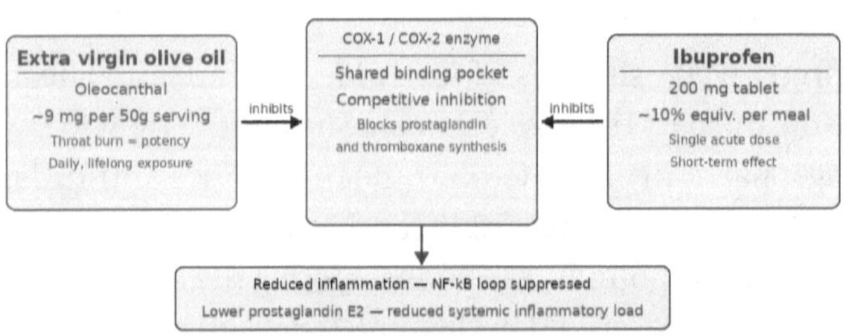

	Oleocanthal (EVOO)	Ibuprofen
Target	COX-1 and COX-2	COX-1 and COX-2
Mechanism	Competitive inhibition	Competitive inhibition
Dose / meal	~9 mg	~200 mg
Frequency	Every meal, lifelong	Acute / episodic

Not a drug — a dietary habit

If your olive oil produces no throat sensation, it contains minimal oleocanthal. The pungent, peppery quality is the pharmacological marker of its anti-inflammatory activity.

FIGURE 8. Oleocanthal and ibuprofen: two compounds sharing one COX enzyme target.

The throat burning is the signal. If your olive oil does not produce any throat sensation when swallowed, it contains minimal oleocanthal — either because it has been refined, because it is old (oleocanthal degrades with time and exposure to light), or because it came from varieties with low phenolic content. The pungent, peppery, throat-catching quality of high-quality fresh extra virgin olive oil is not a flaw — it is the pharmacological marker of its anti-inflammatory activity.

Oleocanthal is not the only anti-inflammatory phenolic in EVOO. Oleuropein (also present in olive leaves), hydroxytyrosol, and tyrosol all contribute to NF-κB suppression through mechanisms including I-kappa-B kinase inhibition and PPAR-gamma activation. EVOO is not a single compound but a pharmacological mixture — which is why olive oil standardized to single phenolic content consistently underperforms whole EVOO in clinical studies.

Omega-3 Fatty Acids: Competing for the Inflammatory Machinery

The cell membranes of every cell in the body contain a mixture of fatty acids. Among these are polyunsaturated fatty acids (PUFAs) that serve as precursors for lipid mediators — prostaglandins, thromboxanes, leukotrienes, and resolvins — that regulate inflammation. The type of PUFA in the membrane determines the type of lipid mediator produced.

Arachidonic acid (AA), an omega-6 PUFA abundant in red meat and refined vegetable oils, is the precursor for pro-inflammatory prostaglandins (PGE2), thromboxane A2 (a platelet aggregation promoter), and leukotriene B4 (a potent neutrophil activator). EPA (eicosapentaenoic acid) and DHA (docosahexaenoic acid), the omega-3 PUFAs from fatty fish, compete with AA for the same COX and LOX enzymes. When EPA and DHA are incorporated into cell membranes, they displace AA and their metabolism produces prostaglandins (PGE3), thromboxanes (TXA3), and leukotrienes (LTB5) that are far less inflammatory than their AA-derived counterparts. EPA and DHA also generate resolvins and protectins — specialized pro-resolving mediators that actively switch off the inflammatory response.[25]

In the context of the T2DM damage network, the most important effects of omega-3 fatty acids are: (1) reduction of NF-κB activation through decreased AA availability and increased resolvin production; (2) direct reduction of DAG accumulation in cell membranes, reducing PKC activation (Chapter 3, Pathway 5); (3) specific protection of the retina, which is uniquely rich in DHA — a fatty acid that must be obtained from diet because the body's conversion from plant-derived ALA is less than 5% efficient.

The ancestral human diet had a ratio near 4:1. The modern Western diet averages 20:1 — a shift that feeds chronic inflammation.

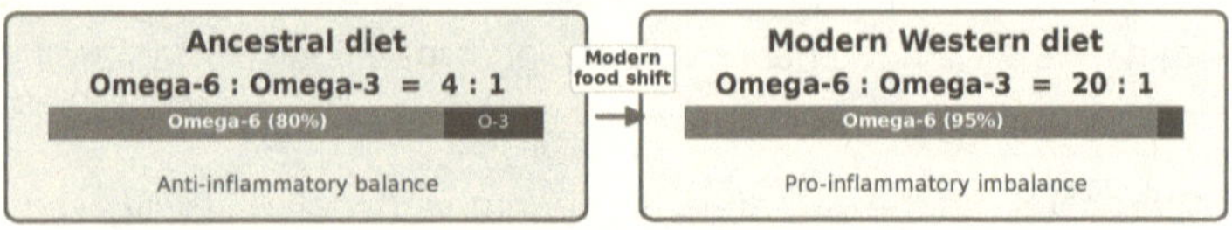

Where each fatty acid comes from

	High omega-6 foods	High omega-3 foods
Main sources	Vegetable oils (corn, soy, sunflower)	Fatty fish (salmon, sardines, mackerel)
Also found in	Processed / fried foods, grain-fed meat	Flaxseed, chia, walnuts (ALA form)
Effect	Drives arachidonic acid → inflammation	EPA/DHA compete with and displace AA

The fix is not a supplement — it is a food swap

EPA and DHA from fatty fish directly compete with arachidonic acid for the same COX and LOX enzymes — displacing the pro-inflammatory substrate at its source. Two servings of fatty fish per week meaningfully shifts the ratio.

FIGURE 9. The omega-6:omega-3 ratio — from ancestral 4:1 to modern Western 20:1

The dose-response relationship is important. The clinical trials showing cardiovascular benefit in high-risk patients used doses of 1 to 4 grams of combined EPA + DHA per day — achievable through 2 to 3 servings per week of fatty fish, or through pharmaceutical-grade omega-3 supplements. The REDUCE-IT trial demonstrated that high-dose icosapentaenoic acid (4 grams/day of EPA alone, as icosapent ethyl) reduced cardiovascular events by 25% in statin-treated patients with elevated triglycerides — many of whom had T2DM. The mechanism appears to involve not only the standard anti-inflammatory EPA effects but specific EPA incorporation into atherosclerotic plaque that stabilizes it against rupture.[26]

Curcumin: The NF-κB Inhibitor in Your Spice Cabinet

Curcumin is the primary polyphenolic pigment in turmeric (Curcuma longa) and the compound responsible for turmeric's deep yellow color. It has been studied more extensively than perhaps any other dietary anti-inflammatory compound, with over 3,000 published studies examining its biological effects. Its primary mechanism relevant to the T2DM damage network is direct inhibition of IKK-beta — the kinase that phosphorylates the NF-κB inhibitor protein I-kappa-B, targeting it for degradation. When IKK-beta is inhibited, I-kappa-B is not degraded, NF-κB remains sequestered in the cytoplasm, and the inflammatory transcription program is not activated.

Curcumin also inhibits RAGE expression (reducing the amplification loop from Chapter 2), activates SIRT1 (opposing the epigenetic memory mechanism from Chapter 4), activates Nrf2 (the master antioxidant transcription factor), and suppresses ER stress through IRE1-alpha inhibition. It is, in effect, a multi-node network suppressor in a single compound.[27]

The clinical evidence in T2DM is substantial. A 2013 randomized controlled trial in patients with prediabetes showed that curcumin supplementation (250mg twice daily of standardized extract) completely prevented progression to T2DM in the treatment group, while 16% of the placebo group progressed. Multiple RCTs in established T2DM have shown improvements in HbA1c (0.4 to 0.8%), fasting glucose, and inflammatory markers.[28]

The critical limitation is bioavailability. Standard curcumin from turmeric powder has oral bioavailability of less than 1%, because it is rapidly metabolized in the gut wall to sulfate and glucuronide conjugates. Two interventions substantially improve bioavailability: (1) piperine, the alkaloid in black pepper, inhibits the gut wall glucuronidation of curcumin and increases its bioavailability by 2,000% — which is why traditional turmeric preparations in Ayurvedic medicine always combine turmeric with black pepper; and (2) lipophilic formulations (curcumin in oil, micellar curcumin, phosphatidylcholine-bound curcumin) exploit curcumin's fat-solubility to bypass the aqueous barrier of the intestinal mucosa.[29]

The PREDIMED Trial and the Mediterranean Pattern

The PREDIMED trial (Prevención con Dieta Mediterránea) enrolled 7,447 high-cardiovascular-risk patients — many with T2DM — and randomized them to Mediterranean diet supplemented with extra virgin olive oil (1 liter per week), Mediterranean diet supplemented with mixed nuts (30g per day), or a control low-fat diet. The trial was stopped early because the olive oil and nut groups had 30% lower rates of major cardiovascular events than the control group — a result so large that continuing the trial was considered unethical.[30]

The mechanism is complex and involves multiple nutrients acting synergistically on multiple network nodes. But the oleocanthal content of the olive oil, the omega-3 fatty acids in the walnuts, and the polyphenols in the olive oil and nuts all contributed to NF-κB suppression through the mechanisms described in this chapter.

WHAT THIS MEANS FOR YOU

THE BOTTOM LINE

The NF-κB inflammatory amplification loop — the self-sustaining cycle that AGEs activate and that eventually runs without elevated glucose — can be partially suppressed through three specific dietary compounds: oleocanthal from high-quality extra virgin olive oil (same mechanism as ibuprofen), EPA and DHA from fatty fish (displacing the pro-inflammatory arachidonic acid from cell membranes), and curcumin from turmeric with black pepper (direct IKK-beta inhibition blocking NF-κB activation). These are not vague anti-inflammatory foods. They are compounds with defined molecular targets in the same network that elevated blood sugar activates.

FOR YOUR PHYSICIAN

Oleocanthal and COX inhibition: Beauchamp GK et al., *Nature* 2005;437:45–46. EVOO polyphenols and NF-κB: Camargo A et al., *J Nutr* 2012;142:1093–1099.

Omega-3 fatty acids and inflammation: Calder PC, *Br J Clin Pharmacol* 2013;75:645–662. REDUCE-IT trial: Bhatt DL et al., *N Engl J Med* 2019;380:11–22. Omega-3 fatty acids and retinal DHA: SanGiovanni JP, Chew EY, *Prog Retin Eye Res* 2005;24:87–138.

Curcumin and NF-κB: Aggarwal BB et al., *Biochem Pharmacol* 2006;71:1397–1421. Curcumin in prediabetes prevention: Chuengsamarn S et al., *Diabetes Care* 2012;35:2121–2127. Piperine bioavailability enhancement: Shoba G et al., *Planta Med* 1998;64:353–356.

PREDIMED trial: Estruch R et al., *N Engl J Med* 2013;368:1279–1290.

CHAPTER 7

Restoring the Antioxidant Defense

Foods That Rebuild NADPH

The antioxidant supplement industry is built on a misconception. For decades, the logic seemed self-evident: oxidative stress damages tissue, antioxidants neutralize oxidants, therefore taking antioxidant vitamins and supplements should reduce oxidative damage. Dozens of large randomized controlled trials tested this hypothesis with vitamins C and E, beta-carotene, and selenium. The results were, to put it charitably, unimpressive — and in several cases, actively harmful.

The reason the logic fails is that it misunderstands how cellular antioxidant defense actually works. The cell does not rely primarily on dietary antioxidants to neutralize reactive oxygen species. It relies on an endogenous antioxidant network — glutathione, superoxide dismutase, catalase, thioredoxin, peroxiredoxins — that is present in every cell and is far more powerful and precisely regulated than any dietary supplement could approximate. Vitamin C and vitamin E play supporting roles in this network, but they are not its primary drivers.

The primary driver is NADPH — nicotinamide adenine dinucleotide phosphate in its reduced form. NADPH is the electron donor that powers glutathione reductase, which regenerates reduced glutathione from its oxidized form. Without NADPH, the entire glutathione system collapses. Vitamin C and vitamin E cannot substitute for it.

As Chapter 3 explained, NADPH production is impaired in T2DM through disruption of the pentose phosphate pathway.

The dietary strategy for this network node is therefore not to supplement antioxidants — it is to restore NADPH production. And the most powerful tool available for doing this is a compound in broccoli sprouts that most people have never heard of.

THE SCIENCE BEHIND THIS

Sulforaphane and the Nrf2 Master Switch

Sulforaphane is an isothiocyanate compound produced when the enzyme myrosinase, present in cruciferous vegetable cells, comes into contact with its substrate glucoraphanin during chewing or chopping. The reaction is a kind of chemical defense system: intact plant cells keep myrosinase and glucoraphanin in separate cellular compartments; when the cell is damaged by a chewing insect or a human jaw, the two compartments mix and sulforaphane is produced.

Sulforaphane is the most potent known dietary activator of a transcription factor called Nrf2 – Nuclear factor erythroid 2-related factor 2. Nrf2 is the master regulator of the cellular antioxidant response. Under normal conditions, Nrf2 is kept in the cytoplasm by a protein called Keap1, which marks Nrf2 for proteasomal degradation. When sulforaphane enters the cell, it chemically modifies specific cysteine residues on Keap1, releasing Nrf2. Free Nrf2 translocates to the nucleus, where it binds to antioxidant response elements (AREs) in the promoters of over 200 cytoprotective genes.[31]

The genes activated by Nrf2 include: glutamate-cysteine ligase (rate-limiting enzyme in glutathione synthesis), glutathione reductase (regenerates NADPH-dependent reduced glutathione), NADPH quinone oxidoreductase (NQO1, reduces quinone radicals), superoxide dismutase, catalase, thioredoxin reductase, and heme oxygenase-1. When sulforaphane activates Nrf2, it simultaneously upregulates the entire antioxidant defense program – not as a one-time surge of electrons from a vitamin pill, but as an upregulation of the cell's own enzymatic defense capacity that persists for hours to days.

The broccoli sprout difference is quantitative and substantial. Three-day-old broccoli sprouts contain 20 to 50 times more glucoraphanin – and therefore more sulforaphane upon myrosinase activation – than mature broccoli. This was established by Paul Talalay's group at Johns Hopkins in 1997, and it has made broccoli sprouts the most sulforaphane-rich dietary source available by a large margin.[32]

The Myrosinase Preservation Problem

Sulforaphane itself is not present in intact broccoli — it is produced when myrosinase acts on glucoraphanin. Heat destroys myrosinase. This means that cooked broccoli has dramatically less sulforaphane production than raw broccoli, even though it contains the same amount of glucoraphanin. A 2011 study by Elizabeth Jeffery showed that steaming broccoli for more than three minutes reduced its sulforaphane yield by over 60%.

There are several practical solutions. First, consuming broccoli sprouts raw preserves myrosinase entirely. Second, when cooking broccoli, adding mustard powder — which contains myrosinase from the mustard seed — to cooked broccoli restores sulforaphane production, because the heat-resistant plant myrosinase in the mustard substitutes for the heat-denatured broccoli myrosinase. Third, eating lightly steamed broccoli (under two minutes) preserves partial myrosinase activity. Fourth, chewing raw broccoli thoroughly before swallowing maximizes myrosinase contact with glucoraphanin.

Riboflavin and the Glutathione Cycle

Glutathione reductase, the enzyme that regenerates reduced glutathione from its oxidized form, requires flavin adenine dinucleotide (FAD) as a cofactor. FAD is derived from riboflavin — vitamin B2. In riboflavin-deficient states, glutathione reductase activity declines and the glutathione cycle slows, impairing NADPH-dependent antioxidant capacity.

Riboflavin deficiency is more common in T2DM patients than in the general population, partly because elevated glucose metabolism increases the demand for B vitamins that serve as cofactors in metabolic pathways. Dietary sources rich in riboflavin include: beef liver (the richest source, not commonly consumed), dairy products, eggs, lean meats, almonds, and dark leafy greens. The daily requirement is 1.1 to 1.3 mg — achievable from dietary sources in most well-nourished patients, but worth reviewing in patients with restricted diets.

Benfotiamine: The Transketolase Activator

Thiamine — vitamin B1 — is the cofactor for transketolase, the enzyme at the junction of the pentose phosphate pathway and glycolysis that can redirect glycolytic byproducts into the PPP rather than into the four damage pathways. In 2003, Hans-Peter Hammes and colleagues published a landmark paper in Nature Medicine showing that benfotiamine — a fat-soluble thiamine derivative that penetrates cell membranes more effectively than water-soluble thiamine

– blocked three of the four major hyperglycemic damage pathways in diabetic rats by activating transketolase and increasing PPP flux. [33]

Benfotiamine is not a standard vitamin B1 supplement. It is a specific synthetic derivative with different absorption and distribution characteristics from thiamine hydrochloride. Clinical trials in diabetic neuropathy have shown that 300 to 600 mg per day of benfotiamine improves nerve conduction velocity and reduces neuropathic pain scores. A 2006 trial by Stracke and colleagues showed that benfotiamine reduces the activation of AGE formation, the polyol pathway, the hexosamine pathway, and PKC simultaneously – by providing transketolase with adequate cofactor to redirect the triose phosphate intermediates that would otherwise fuel these pathways. [34]

Growing Your Own Broccoli Sprouts

Broccoli sprouts are available in some specialty grocery stores but are expensive and not universally accessible. Growing them at home is straightforward, inexpensive, and requires no soil or special equipment. The protocol: (1) Obtain organic broccoli sprouting seeds – not broccoli floret seeds, which do not produce the same glucoraphanin content. (2) Soak one tablespoon of seeds in water for 8 hours. (3) Drain, rinse, and place in a jar with a mesh or cheesecloth lid. (4) Rinse and drain twice daily for 3 days. (5) Spread in indirect light on day 3 for 4 to 6 hours to initiate chlorophyll production. (6) Eat. The 3-day sprouts are the sulforaphane peak – after day 5, glucoraphanin content begins to decline as the plant metabolizes it. One tablespoon of seeds produces approximately 100 grams of sprouts, enough for one serving.

WHAT THIS MEANS FOR YOU

THE BOTTOM LINE

The cellular antioxidant defense system runs on NADPH, not on vitamin supplements. The most powerful dietary intervention for NADPH production is sulforaphane from broccoli sprouts, which activates the Nrf2 master switch and simultaneously upregulates glutathione synthesis, glutathione reductase, superoxide dismutase, catalase, and over 200 other cytoprotective genes. Three-day-old broccoli sprouts contain 20 to 50 times more sulforaphane precursor than mature broccoli. Growing them at home takes three days and requires nothing but seeds, a jar, and water.

FOR YOUR PHYSICIAN

Broccoli sprout sulforaphane content: Fahey JW et al., *PNAS* 1997;94:10367–10372. Nrf2 as master antioxidant regulator: Itoh K et al., *Mol Cell Biol* 1997;17:1502–1509.

Cooking and myrosinase inactivation: Jeffery EH, Araya M, *Phytochem Rev* 2009;8:309–324. Mustard powder restoration: Vermeulen M et al., *Mol Nutr Food Res* 2008;52:1047–1057.

Benfotiamine blocking hyperglycemic damage pathways: Hammes HP et al., *Nat Med* 2003;9:294–299. Benfotiamine in diabetic neuropathy: Stracke H et al., *Exp Clin Endocrinol Diabetes* 2008;116:600–605.

CHAPTER 8

The Sorbitol Trap

Foods That Protect Your Nerves and Eyes

Thomas has had T2DM for nine years. At his last ophthalmology appointment, he was told his lenses are developing early nuclear sclerosis — the beginning of diabetic cataract. His monofilament exam shows reduced sensation in three toes. His neurologist has noted slowing in nerve conduction velocity. His kidneys are fine, his retina is fine, and his HbA1c has been consistently around 7.9%.

The pattern is characteristic: Thomas's damage is concentrated in the tissues where glucose entry does not require insulin and therefore rises in proportion to blood sugar — the lens of the eye, the peripheral nerves, the kidney tubules. These are the tissues of the polyol pathway, and the compounds discussed in this chapter specifically target the enzyme that initiates it.

Aldose reductase — the enzyme that converts glucose to sorbitol — has been a pharmaceutical target for over forty years. Drug companies have invested enormous resources in synthetic aldose reductase inhibitors, and several have reached Phase III clinical trials. None has succeeded well enough to reach approval in major Western markets, primarily because of toxicity issues and because the clinical trials were conducted in patients with already-established complications, where preventing accumulation of further damage is a weaker endpoint than reversing existing damage.

Nature, however, has produced several aldose reductase inhibitors that are present in food in meaningful concentrations, have excellent safety profiles, and can be consumed daily for a lifetime without concern. The most important of these is quercetin.

THE SCIENCE BEHIND THIS

Quercetin: The Aldose Reductase Inhibitor in Your Kitchen

Quercetin is a flavonol — a subclass of flavonoids — found in a wide range of plant foods. It is one of the most abundant dietary polyphenols consumed globally, and it has been studied more extensively than almost any other flavonoid. Its structural interaction with the aldose reductase active site was described in detail in the 1980s by Costantino and colleagues, who showed that quercetin fits into the enzyme's active site in a manner that blocks glucose binding, reducing catalytic activity by approximately 65% at concentrations achievable in human tissues with regular dietary intake.[35]

The foods with the highest quercetin content per 100 grams, in descending order: capers (234 mg/100g raw), lovage leaves (170 mg/100g), radish leaves (70 mg/100g), carob (58 mg/100g), dill (55 mg/100g), coriander leaf (53 mg/100g), red onion (35 mg/100g), white onion (20 mg/100g), apples with skin (4.4 mg/100g), and broccoli (3.4 mg/100g). The difference between capers and apples is striking: capers contain over 50 times the quercetin of apples. They are not a common dietary staple in most Western countries, but they are inexpensive, shelf-stable, and can be added to salads, pasta sauces, and egg preparations without significantly altering the flavor profile of a meal.

Red onions contain approximately 75% more quercetin than white or yellow onions, and the quercetin is concentrated in the outer layers of the onion — which most cooks discard. Cooking in water with onion skins included (for soups and broths) extracts the quercetin into the cooking liquid. The quercetin in onions is present primarily as quercetin glucoside, which is absorbed somewhat less efficiently than the aglycone form — but the large amounts in red onion still provide meaningful intake.

The Lens Protection Argument

The evidence for quercetin's protection of the eye lens from sorbitol accumulation is particularly compelling because the lens provides a nearly ideal experimental model: it is avascular (no blood supply), it maintains glucose concentrations in direct proportion to plasma glucose, and cataract formation can be precisely quantified. In organ culture studies, human lens tissue incubated in high-glucose conditions develops opacity that is substantially reduced by quercetin at physiologically achievable concentrations. The mechanism is aldose reductase inhibition reducing sorbitol accumulation and the consequent osmotic disruption of crystallin protein arrangement.[36]

Resveratrol's Role in the Polyol Pathway

Resveratrol — the stilbene polyphenol from red grapes, blueberries, and peanuts — has a secondary aldose reductase inhibitory effect in addition to its primary SIRT1-activating role described in Chapter 4. It also activates the glyoxalase I enzyme (the methylglyoxal detox enzyme described in Chapter 2), providing additional benefit to the polyol pathway node by reducing the methylglyoxal that AGEs from the polyol pathway would otherwise generate.[37]

Resveratrol's bioavailability from food sources is low — the amounts in red wine and blueberries are insufficient to produce the tissue concentrations that in vitro studies suggest are needed for significant aldose reductase inhibition. This is an area where supplementation may be more appropriate than food-only intake. Micronized resveratrol preparations (which reduce particle size to improve absorption) and pterostilbene (a methylated resveratrol analog with higher bioavailability and longer half-life) are reasonable supplemental options for patients specifically concerned about neuropathy or cataract protection.

Luteolin and Kaempferol: Supporting Flavonols

Two other dietary flavonols with meaningful aldose reductase inhibitory activity are luteolin and kaempferol. Luteolin is found at highest concentrations in fresh thyme (564 mg/100g), dried oregano (1028 mg/100g — the highest luteolin content of any food), celery seeds, and peppers. Kaempferol is abundant in capers (alongside quercetin), kale, broccoli, leeks, chives, and green beans.

These flavonols interact with the same aldose reductase active site as quercetin, and their combined effect when consumed together from mixed plant sources may be additive. This provides a mechanistic rationale for dietary diversity as a strategy for polyol pathway suppression: a diet that regularly includes red onion, capers, fresh herbs, broccoli, and dark leafy greens delivers multiple aldose reductase inhibitors simultaneously.

WHAT THIS MEANS FOR YOU

THE BOTTOM LINE

The polyol pathway converts glucose to sorbitol in the tissues that are least protected by insulin – the lens of the eye, the peripheral nerves, the kidney tubules. Sorbitol cannot leave the cells, causes osmotic damage, and depletes the NADPH that powers antioxidant defense. Quercetin, the flavonol most abundant in capers and red onions, inhibits aldose reductase – the enzyme that initiates this pathway – by approximately 65% at concentrations achievable through regular dietary intake. Two tablespoons of capers deliver more quercetin than most people consume from all food sources in a day.

FOR YOUR PHYSICIAN

Quercetin as aldose reductase inhibitor: Costantino L et al., *J Med Chem* 1999;42:1881–1893.
Quercetin content of foods: USDA Flavonoid Database.
Quercetin and lens cataract protection: Gong X, Shang F, *J Nutr* 2009;139:1567–1572.
Resveratrol and glyoxalase I activation: Xue M et al., *Diabetes* 2014;63:3914–3925.

CHAPTER 9

The Insulin Resistance Amplifier

Breaking the Hexosamine Cycle

The hexosamine pathway presents a particularly insidious challenge: it is a vicious cycle. The more glucose that flows through it, the more O-GlcNAc modification accumulates on insulin signaling proteins, the worse insulin resistance becomes, the higher blood sugar rises, the more glucose flows through the pathway. Chapter 3 described this molecular mechanism. This chapter addresses it with the most evidence-based dietary supplement for type 2 diabetes available.[38]

Berberine is not a household name. It should be. It is a yellow alkaloid found in the roots and bark of several plants — Berberis vulgaris (barberry), Berberis aristata, Coptis chinensis (goldenseal's Chinese relative), and Hydrastis canadensis (goldenseal). It has been used in traditional Chinese and Ayurvedic medicine for centuries, primarily as an antimicrobial agent for gastrointestinal infections. In 2006, researchers at Shanghai's Jiao Tong University discovered something that changed berberine's status entirely: it activates AMPK through the same mechanism as metformin, and in randomized controlled trials, it reduces HbA1c by nearly as much as metformin in head-to-head comparisons.

THE SCIENCE BEHIND THIS

Berberine: The AMPK Activator in a Plant

AMPK — AMP-activated protein kinase — is the cell's master energy sensor. When ATP (the cell's energy currency) is depleted and AMP accumulates, AMPK is activated. Its activation triggers a cascade of responses designed to restore energy balance: it increases glucose uptake in muscle cells, activates fatty acid oxidation, inhibits fatty acid and cholesterol synthesis, and — most relevant to the hexosamine pathway — reduces glucose flux through non-glycolytic side pathways by directing glucose toward ATP-producing pathways.

Metformin's primary mechanism of action is inhibition of mitochondrial Complex I, which reduces ATP production slightly, raises the AMP/ATP ratio, and activates AMPK. This is why metformin's main side effect is gastrointestinal — the same Complex I inhibition that activates AMPK in hepatocytes also affects the intestinal epithelium at standard doses.

Berberine inhibits mitochondrial Complex I through a structurally similar mechanism to metformin, activating AMPK through the same AMP/ATP sensing pathway. In a 2006 randomized controlled trial by Yin and colleagues, berberine 500mg three times daily reduced fasting glucose by 36%, postprandial glucose by 44%, HbA1c by 2.0%, and triglycerides by 35.9% in patients with newly diagnosed T2DM — results comparable to those achieved by metformin in the same study.[39]

Fourteen subsequent RCTs have confirmed the glucose-lowering effect of berberine, with a consistent HbA1c reduction of 0.9 to 1.2% versus placebo in T2DM patients. A 2012 Cochrane-style meta-analysis of 14 trials concluded that berberine combined with lifestyle intervention reduced HbA1c more than lifestyle intervention alone, and that berberine plus oral hypoglycemic agents reduced HbA1c more than oral hypoglycemics alone.[40]

Berberine's Multi-Node Network Effects

Beyond its AMPK-mediated glucose lowering, berberine addresses multiple nodes of the damage network simultaneously. It activates SIRT1 through AMPK-dependent NAD+ elevation, opposing the epigenetic memory mechanism. It reduces hexosamine pathway flux by directing glucose toward ATP-producing metabolism rather than the side pathway. It activates the glyoxalase I enzyme, reducing methylglyoxal accumulation. It induces GLP-1 secretion from intestinal L-cells (and, as Chapter 20 will describe, it also activates gut

TAS2R bitter receptors). It reduces inflammatory cytokine production through NF-κB inhibition. And it has specific hepatic effects — reducing hepatic glucose output through AMPK-mediated inhibition of gluconeogenic enzymes — that complement metformin's mechanism.

Berberine also modifies the gut microbiome in ways that may contribute to its metabolic effects: it selectively increases Akkermansia muciniphila and Bifidobacterium species, the bacteria most associated with healthy metabolic function, while reducing the gram-negative bacteria whose lipopolysaccharide contributes to systemic inflammation.

The Carbohydrate Restriction Mechanism

The most direct dietary intervention on the hexosamine pathway is simply to reduce the total glucose flux through glycolysis — which means reducing carbohydrate intake, particularly refined carbohydrate that is rapidly absorbed and produces large glucose spikes. The hexosamine pathway typically handles 2 to 3% of normal glucose flux; in hyperglycemia, this fraction increases substantially because the pathway's rate-limiting enzyme (glutamine:fructose-6-phosphate amidotransferase, GFAT) becomes saturated.

Low-carbohydrate dietary patterns — reducing carbohydrate intake to 50 to 130 grams per day, without necessarily reaching ketogenic levels — consistently reduce fasting insulin, HOMA-IR, and postprandial glucose spikes. These improvements in insulin sensitivity are attributable, at least in part, to reduced hexosamine pathway activity and decreased O-GlcNAc modification of IRS-1 and Akt.

The glycemic hierarchy of Chapter 5 is the practical framework for this reduction: by choosing lower-GL carbohydrates, increasing resistant starch consumption, eating protein and vegetables before carbohydrates, and using soluble fiber as a glucose absorption moderator, most patients can substantially reduce their effective carbohydrate load without eliminating carbohydrates from their diet.

Cinnamon: A Modest but Real Hexosamine Pathway Effect

Cinnamon (specifically Cinnamomum verum — Ceylon cinnamon, not the more common Cassia cinnamon) contains polyphenolic polymers called type A proanthocyanidins that activate insulin receptor tyrosine kinase, mimic the post-receptor insulin signaling cascade, and reduce O-GlcNAc modification of insulin signaling proteins. A 2003 RCT by Khan and colleagues showed that 1 to 6 grams of Cassia cinnamon per day reduced fasting glucose by 18 to

29% in Pakistani T2DM patients. Subsequent meta-analyses have shown more modest effects (fasting glucose reduction of 10 to 29 mg/dL) with considerable trial heterogeneity.[41]

The important caveat is the cinnamon species distinction. Cassia cinnamon (the variety sold in most Western supermarkets) contains significant amounts of coumarin, a natural compound that is hepatotoxic at high doses. The European Food Safety Authority has established a tolerable daily intake of 0.1 mg/kg body weight for coumarin, which limits safe Cassia cinnamon consumption to about half a teaspoon per day for most adults. Ceylon cinnamon (available in specialty stores and online) contains negligible coumarin and can be used more freely. If using cinnamon for its metabolic effects, choose Ceylon cinnamon or use standardized cinnamon extract supplements.

WHAT THIS MEANS FOR YOU

THE BOTTOM LINE

The hexosamine pathway converts a small fraction of glucose into a signaling molecule that modifies insulin receptor proteins and makes insulin resistance progressively worse. Breaking this vicious cycle requires reducing glucose flux through the pathway — achieved through carbohydrate quality (lower GL foods), carbohydrate quantity (moderate restriction to 100 to 130g net carbs), and AMPK activation. Berberine activates AMPK through the same mechanism as metformin and reduces HbA1c by 0.9 to 1.2% in randomized controlled trials — making it the most evidence-based dietary supplement for T2DM currently available.

FOR YOUR PHYSICIAN

Berberine's AMPK activation mechanism: Hawley SA et al., *J Biol Chem* 2010;285:28109–28117. Initial berberine RCT vs metformin: Yin J et al., *Metabolism* 2008;57:712–717. Meta-analysis of berberine in T2DM: Dong H et al., *Evid Based Complement Alternat Med* 2012;2012:591654.

Hexosamine pathway and insulin resistance: Hart GW et al., *Annu Rev Biochem* 2011;80:825–858.

Cinnamon and insulin sensitization: Khan A et al., *Diabetes Care* 2003;26:3215–3218. Coumarin in Cassia cinnamon: European Food Safety Authority, *EFSA J* 2008;793:1–15.

CHAPTER 10

Protecting the Blood Vessels

Omega-3s, PKC, and the Heart

The cardiovascular complications of T2DM are not simply the consequence of blocked arteries. They are the consequence of a biological process that begins in the cell membrane — in the specific fatty acids that make up that membrane, in the lipid signals those fatty acids produce, and in the protein kinase that those signals activate.

Chapter 3 introduced the protein kinase C pathway: how diacylglycerol accumulates in hyperglycemic cells and activates PKC, which drives VEGF in the retina, fibrosis in the kidney, and endothelial dysfunction throughout the vasculature. This chapter describes in detail how omega-3 fatty acids suppress this pathway at its origin — not by blocking an enzyme downstream, but by changing the composition of the cell membrane so that the signal molecule (DAG) is never produced in the first place.

THE SCIENCE BEHIND THIS

Cell Membrane Composition as a Therapeutic Target

Cell membranes are not passive barriers. They are dynamic, fluid structures whose composition determines which signals can be generated within them and which cannot. Phospholipids – the building blocks of cell membranes – contain a glycerol backbone with two fatty acid chains attached. The fatty acid composition of cell membrane phospholipids reflects, with a lag of weeks to months, the fatty acid composition of the diet.

Arachidonic acid (AA), the omega-6 PUFA most associated with pro-inflammatory signaling, is esterified into cell membrane phospholipids.

When phospholipase C cleaves membrane phospholipids in response to cellular signals, it releases diacylglycerol (DAG) containing AA. This DAG activates PKC-beta. PKC-beta phosphorylates VEGFR2 in retinal endothelial cells, amplifying VEGF signaling. PKC-beta phosphorylates eNOS at an inhibitory site, reducing nitric oxide production. PKC-beta activates TGF-beta in glomerular mesangial cells, driving the fibrosis that thickens the glomerular basement membrane.

When EPA and DHA from fatty fish are incorporated into cell membrane phospholipids — which occurs over weeks to months of regular fish consumption — they partially displace AA. When phospholipase C now cleaves these phospholipids, the DAG produced contains EPA and DHA rather than AA. This DAG activates PKC far less potently than AA-containing DAG, because EPA and DHA produce resolvins and protectins rather than the pro-inflammatory prostaglandins and thromboxanes that AA produces.

This is membrane pharmacology: changing the substrate for PKC activation by changing the membrane composition. It is one of the most elegant examples in nutritional medicine of a dietary intervention that works by reshaping the molecular environment rather than blocking an enzyme.

The Retinal DHA Argument

The retina is the most DHA-rich tissue in the body. Photoreceptor outer segment membranes contain the highest concentration of DHA of any tissue — approximately 50% of their phospholipid fatty acids. DHA in the retina is not there by accident: it is actively concentrated there by specific transport proteins because it is essential for photoreceptor function. The fluidity and curvature of DHA-rich membranes facilitates the conformational changes of rhodopsin that convert light into neural signals.[42]

DHA must be obtained from diet, because the body's enzymatic conversion of plant-derived ALA to DHA is less than 5% efficient. Patients who consume little fatty fish and take no DHA supplement have DHA-depleted retinal membranes, and retinal AA is higher relative to DHA. This shifts the membrane PKC activation substrate toward AA-derived DAG, increasing PKC-beta activity in retinal vascular cells.

Multiple prospective epidemiological studies have shown that higher dietary omega-3 intake is associated with slower progression of diabetic retinopathy. The PREDIMED trial sub-analysis showed that the Mediterranean diet with added EVOO (which included significant fish consumption) reduced diabetic retinopathy progression. The OPTIC trial and related studies suggest that omega-3 supplementation reduces diabetic macular edema severity.[43]

The Triglyceride-Lowering Effect and Its Network Relevance

Omega-3 fatty acids at doses of 2 to 4 grams per day consistently reduce fasting triglycerides by 25 to 50% — one of the most potent triglyceride-lowering interventions available without a prescription. This is relevant to the damage network because hypertriglyceridemia is associated with elevated DAG production in vascular cells (from TG-rich lipoprotein hydrolysis), additional PKC activation, and progression of endothelial dysfunction.

The mechanism of omega-3 triglyceride lowering is primarily hepatic: EPA and DHA reduce hepatic VLDL secretion by inhibiting the diacylglycerol acyltransferase enzyme that incorporates DAG into triglycerides. This same enzyme inhibition reduces hepatic DAG availability for PKC activation.

Beyond the Heart: Omega-3s and the Nervous System

DHA is the dominant fatty acid not only in the retina but in neuronal cell membranes throughout the central and peripheral nervous system. DHA-rich neuronal membranes support faster axonal conduction, better synaptic vesicle release, and more effective long-term potentiation. In the context of diabetic peripheral neuropathy, DHA depletion in Schwann cell membranes may contribute to the slowed nerve conduction velocity characteristic of the condition.

A 2018 RCT by Lewis and colleagues showed that omega-3 supplementation (four grams per day for 12 months) improved small fiber regeneration in patients with diabetic peripheral neuropathy — a finding consistent with the role of DHA in axonal membrane composition. The effect was modest but statistically significant and mechanistically plausible.[44]

WHAT THIS MEANS FOR YOU

THE BOTTOM LINE

Omega-3 fatty acids EPA and DHA suppress the PKC pathway by incorporating into cell membranes and displacing the arachidonic acid that is the source of the PKC-activating diacylglycerol signal. This is not a downstream enzyme blockade – it is a change in membrane composition that prevents the activating signal from being generated. DHA must be obtained from diet because the body's conversion from plant sources is less than 5% efficient. The retina is particularly DHA-dependent, and DHA depletion in retinal cell membranes increases PKC-beta activation and VEGF-driven vessel damage.

FOR YOUR PHYSICIAN

Omega-3 membrane incorporation and PKC: Siddiqui RA et al., *Prostaglandins Leukot Essent Fatty Acids* 2008;78:301–316. EPA/DHA and VEGF reduction: Koto T et al. *Invest Ophthalmol Vis Sci* 2007;48:155–163.

Omega-3 and diabetic retinopathy: SanGiovanni JP, Chew EY, *Prog Retin Eye Res* 2005;24:87–138. PREDIMED retinopathy sub-analysis: Sala-Vila A et al., *JAMA Ophthalmol* 2016;134:1142–1149.

Omega-3 and diabetic neuropathy: Lewis EJ et al., *J Diabetes Investig* 2018;9:1455–1462.

REDUCE-IT: Bhatt DL et al., *N Engl J Med* 2019;380:11–22.

CHAPTER 11

Calming the Protein Factory

Foods That Reduce ER Stress

There is a cellular catastrophe that unfolds slowly, silently, and without symptoms in the pancreatic beta cells of patients with long-standing T2DM. Inside those cells, the endoplasmic reticulum — the protein synthesis factory described in Chapter 3 — is overwhelmed. The combination of AGE-modified proteins that cannot be properly folded, the disrupted ER membrane caused by lipid dysregulation, and the calcium channel dysfunction from oxidative stress has created a protein folding crisis from which the cell cannot recover.

The unfolded protein response — the alarm system the ER activates when folding demand exceeds capacity — has been running in a chronic state for years. In this state, one of its branches activates a protein called CHOP. CHOP kills cells. Beta cells that have activated CHOP-driven apoptosis do not regenerate. The progressive beta cell loss that accelerates the transition from early T2DM to insulin-requiring T2DM is, in significant part, the consequence of chronic ER stress in the islets of Langerhans.[45]

This chapter describes dietary interventions that reduce the ER's protein-folding burden — the chemical chaperones and direct UPR modulators that are the most mechanistically novel dietary targets in the book. It also describes the compound from green tea that has the strongest direct evidence for ER stress reduction: EGCG.

THE SCIENCE BEHIND THIS

EGCG: The Green Tea Polyphenol that Quiets the UPR

Epigallocatechin gallate (EGCG) is the most abundant catechin in green tea, comprising 50 to 80% of the catechin content. A standard cup of green tea (2 grams of tea leaves in 200 mL hot water, steeped for three minutes) contains approximately 100 to 150 mg of EGCG. A cup of matcha prepared from powdered whole tea leaves contains approximately 300 to 450 mg of EGCG.

EGCG's anti-diabetic mechanisms are multiple. It activates AMPK, contributing to the same insulin-sensitizing pathway as berberine and metformin. It activates SIRT1, opposing the epigenetic memory mechanism of Chapter 4. It inhibits glucosidases, reducing carbohydrate digestion speed (a mild dietary acarbose effect). But its most novel and mechanistically compelling effect in the context of ER stress is its inhibition of IRE1-alpha — one of the three ER stress sensors described in Chapter 3.

IRE1-alpha is the ER stress sensor responsible for activating the JNK signaling pathway that impairs IRS-1 function and worsens insulin resistance. It is also responsible for generating the inflammatory signal from the ER stress response that contributes to NF-κB activation. When EGCG inhibits IRE1-alpha, it simultaneously reduces ER stress-driven insulin resistance, ER stress-driven inflammation, and ER stress-driven CHOP activation (which occurs through the PERK branch that IRE1-alpha amplifies).

A 2017 RCT by Liu and colleagues showed that green tea extract supplementation (500mg per day of EGCG-standardized extract) over 12 weeks reduced fasting glucose, fasting insulin, HOMA-IR, and hs-CRP in overweight patients with insulin resistance. The reduction in HOMA-IR (25%) is consistent with a mechanism that includes ER stress reduction, not just AMPK activation.[46]

The Chemical Chaperone Concept

A chemical chaperone is a small molecule that stabilizes protein conformation, reducing the tendency of proteins to misfold in the first place and thereby reducing the load on the ER's protein folding machinery. The most potent chemical chaperone studied in the context of T2DM is tauroursodeoxycholic acid (TUDCA) — a bile acid derivative that is produced endogenously in the liver and is also present in small amounts in some fermented foods (particularly fermented soy products).

Intravenous TUDCA was shown by Bhatt and colleagues at Harvard in 2011 to reduce hepatic and muscle insulin resistance in obese patients with insulin resistance, with mechanisms including ER stress reduction in hepatocytes and skeletal muscle cells. Oral TUDCA supplementation at 1,750 mg per day reproduced these effects in a subsequent RCT. The mechanism is direct stabilization of nascent proteins in the ER lumen, reducing the accumulation of misfolded proteins that trigger the UPR.[47]

TUDCA is available as a supplement at 250 to 500 mg capsules and is commercially produced through bacterial biotransformation. It is not present in food at therapeutically meaningful concentrations. It should be considered a pharmaceutical-grade supplement rather than a dietary intervention — with meaningful mechanistic rationale and limited but suggestive clinical trial data. It is appropriate for discussion with a physician before use, rather than for routine supplementation.

Curcumin's ER Stress Effect

Chapter 6 introduced curcumin primarily as an NF-κB inhibitor through IKK-beta blockade. It also addresses ER stress through a separate mechanism: curcumin inhibits IRE1-alpha's kinase activity (similar to EGCG), reduces the expression of GRP78 (the ER chaperone that marks stress severity) at high activation states, and activates the heat shock response that upregulates molecular chaperones including HSP70 and HSP90.

The NASH evidence for curcumin is particularly relevant here: NASH (non-alcoholic steatohepatitis) involves hepatic ER stress as a central mechanism, and curcumin's histological benefit in NASH demonstrated in the PIVENS trial and subsequent studies is consistent with its ER stress-reducing properties. For T2DM patients with concomitant fatty liver disease — a very common combination — curcumin's combined NF-κB and ER stress effects make it the most multi-mechanistic single compound in the dietary pharmacology of T2DM.

NAD+ and the ER-Mitochondria Connection

The mitochondria-associated membrane (MAM) — the physical junction between the ER and the mitochondria — is a critical site of calcium transfer between the two organelles. Adequate calcium transfer from the ER to the mitochondria is required for optimal mitochondrial ATP production and for the maintenance of ER calcium stores (which are needed by the calcium-dependent ER chaperones). When NAD+ is depleted by the NF-κB-PARP pathway described in Chapter 4, mitochondrial function declines, MAM integrity deteriorates, and ER calcium homeostasis is disrupted — which worsens ER stress.

This connection provides a mechanistic rationale for NAD+ precursor supplementation in the context of ER stress: maintaining adequate NAD+ levels supports both SIRT1 activity (epigenetic protection) and mitochondrial function (ER calcium homeostasis). Nicotinamide riboside and NMN are the precursors with the best evidence for raising intracellular NAD+ levels in humans.

WHAT THIS MEANS FOR YOU

THE BOTTOM LINE

The endoplasmic reticulum stress response is the molecular mechanism through which the protein factory of the cell declares a crisis — and its chronic activation in T2DM drives progressive beta-cell death, worsening insulin resistance, and amplified NF-κB inflammation. EGCG from green tea (2 to 4 cups per day, or matcha) inhibits IRE1-alpha, the ER stress sensor that drives insulin resistance and inflammation. Curcumin addresses ER stress through a complementary pathway. TUDCA, the chemical chaperone, directly reduces protein misfolding burden. These interventions protect the beta cells that your body needs to maintain whatever endogenous insulin secretion remains.

FOR YOUR PHYSICIAN

EGCG and IRE1-alpha inhibition: Zhao D et al., *Biochem Biophys Res Commun* 2017;490:155–162. EGCG RCT in insulin resistance: Liu CY et al., *J Nutr* 2014;144:491–500.

TUDCA and insulin resistance: Bhatt DL et al., *J Clin Endocrinol Metab* 2011;96:E995–E999. Oral TUDCA trial: Kars M et al., *Diabetes* 2010;59:3375–3381.

Curcumin and ER stress: Zhao LN et al., *Eur J Pharmacol* 2020;887:173575.

ER stress and beta-cell apoptosis via CHOP: Oyadomari S et al., *J Clin Invest* 2002;109:525–532.

Closing Reflection on Part II

Part II has addressed each of the seven network nodes with specific, evidence-based dietary interventions. The connections can be summarized as follows:

The glycation cascade (GCN node): Reduce dietary AGEs through moist-heat cooking and acidic marinades (Chapter 1). Reduce blood glucose spikes through glycemic load management, resistant starch, meal sequencing, and soluble fiber (Chapter 5).

The inflammatory amplifier (NF-κB): Oleocanthal from extra virgin olive oil, EPA/DHA from fatty fish, curcumin with black pepper (Chapter 6).

The antioxidant defense (PPP node): Sulforaphane from broccoli sprouts via Nrf2 activation, riboflavin for glutathione reductase, benfotiamine for transketolase and PPP flux restoration (Chapter 7).

The sorbitol trap (POL node): Quercetin from capers and red onions, resveratrol and pterostilbene for aldose reductase inhibition and glyoxalase I activation (Chapter 8).

The insulin resistance amplifier (HBP node): Berberine for AMPK activation and hexosamine pathway flux reduction, carbohydrate quality management, Ceylon cinnamon (Chapter 9).

The blood vessel damage driver (PKC node): EPA and DHA membrane incorporation from fatty fish, reduction of omega-6 refined oils (Chapter 10).

The protein factory crisis (UPR node): EGCG from green tea for IRE1-alpha inhibition, curcumin for complementary ER stress reduction, TUDCA as a chemical chaperone (Chapter 11).

No single food, supplement, or dietary pattern addresses all seven nodes simultaneously. The dietary strategy that comes closest is the one that underlies every recommendation in this part: a Mediterranean-style eating pattern rich in fatty fish, extra virgin olive oil, cruciferous vegetables, quercetin-rich onions and capers, green tea, turmeric with black pepper, and legumes — with controlled carbohydrate quality, meal sequencing, and resistant starch from cooled and reheated grains. This pattern is not a coincidence. It represents thousands of years of empirical convergence on the same molecular targets that modern biochemistry has identified as the nodes of the damage network.

Part III now turns from the biology of food to the arithmetic of eating: how many calories, how many grams of carbohydrate, and how to build a plate that delivers every principle in Parts I and II in a form that is practical, sustainable, and genuinely enjoyable.

Part III

The Numbers You Need to Know

Caloric need, carbohydrate load, glycemic index, portion construction.The mathematics of eating for T2DM made accessible and actionable.

Parts I and II gave you the biology: what elevated blood sugar does to your tissues, and which foods suppress which nodes of the damage network. Part III gives you the arithmetic: how many calories your body actually needs, how to think about carbohydrate in a way that is both accurate and practical, and how to construct a plate that delivers every principle of Parts I and II in a format you can sustain for a lifetime.

These three chapters are the most practical in the book. They contain tables, calculations, and specific numbers. Readers who prefer not to engage with arithmetic can focus on the practical boxes and the bottom lines and still leave with a workable framework. Readers who want to understand the numbers precisely — as their physician does — will find the calculations fully explained.

One important caution before we begin: the numbers in this part are starting points, not prescriptions. Human metabolism varies substantially between individuals, and the calculations here produce estimates that may be off by 10 to 20% in either direction for any specific person. The right way to use these numbers is to start with the calculation, implement for four to six weeks, observe what happens to body weight and blood sugar, and adjust accordingly. The mathematics is a map, not a destination.

CHAPTER 12

How Many Calories Does Your Body Actually Need?

Elena is fifty-two years old, five feet four inches tall, weighs 178 pounds, and works as a high school teacher — on her feet for most of the school day but not engaging in deliberate exercise. She has had T2DM for six years, and her physician has recommended that she lose 20 pounds. Elena has tried three different calorie-restricted diets in the past four years, all of which produced initial weight loss followed by a plateau and eventual regain. She is not sure how many calories she should be eating, and every number she has read online seems different.

Elena's frustration is valid, and it has a specific cause: most calorie estimates she has encountered were calculated for a generic "average adult" rather than for her. A fifty-two-year-old woman with T2DM, insulin resistance, and a moderately active lifestyle has specific metabolic characteristics that differ from the average adult in ways that matter for caloric calculation.

This chapter walks through the calculation step by step, using Elena as a worked example, and then provides a framework you can apply to your own situation.

THE SCIENCE BEHIND THIS

Resting Metabolic Rate: The Foundation of Everything

Your resting metabolic rate (RMR) — sometimes called basal metabolic rate (BMR) — is the number of calories your body burns at complete rest over 24 hours just to maintain vital functions: breathing, heartbeat, body temperature, brain function, cell repair, and the constant work of maintaining ionic gradients across cell membranes. It accounts for 60 to 70% of total daily energy expenditure for most sedentary to lightly active people.

The most accurate equation for estimating RMR in clinical practice is the Mifflin-St Jeor equation, published in 1990 and validated across diverse populations:[48]

For women: RMR (kcal/day) = (10 × weight in kg) + (6.25 × height in cm) - (5 × age in years) - 161

For men: RMR (kcal/day) = (10 × weight in kg) + (6.25 × height in cm) - (5 × age in years) + 5

For Elena (52 years, 80.7 kg, 162.6 cm):

RMR = (10 × 80.7) + (6.25 × 162.6) - (5 × 52) - 161

RMR = 807 + 1016 - 260 - 161 = 1,402 kcal/day

This is the number of calories Elena's body burns every day doing nothing. She cannot eat fewer than this without suppressing vital metabolic functions. It is her floor, not her target.

The Activity Multiplier: From Resting to Living

To estimate total daily energy expenditure (TDEE) — the actual number of calories Elena burns going through her day — her RMR is multiplied by an activity factor:

Sedentary (desk job, no deliberate exercise): RMR × 1.2

Lightly active (light exercise 1–3 days/week, or on feet at work like Elena): RMR × 1.375

Moderately active (exercise 3–5 days/week): RMR × 1.55

Very active (hard exercise 6–7 days/week): RMR × 1.725

Extra active (physical job + hard daily exercise): RMR × 1.9

For Elena (lightly active, on her feet at work):

TDEE = 1,402 × 1.375 = 1,928 kcal/day

This is Elena's maintenance caloric intake: the number of calories she needs to eat each day to maintain her current weight. To lose weight, she needs to eat less than this.

The T2DM Adjustment: Why Standard Calculations Slightly Overestimate

Patients with T2DM and significant insulin resistance have two metabolic characteristics that slightly reduce their effective TDEE compared to the standard calculation. First, insulin resistance impairs the uptake and utilization of glucose in muscle and adipose tissue, meaning that a portion of dietary glucose is less efficiently converted to energy (some is excreted in urine as glycosuria, and some drives lipogenesis in the liver rather than muscle ATP production). Second, the elevated insulin levels of hyperinsulinemia suppress fat oxidation, meaning that even when caloric intake slightly exceeds the calculation, fat burning is reduced and weight gain occurs more readily than in insulin-sensitive individuals.

In practice, this means that T2DM patients often need to eat 5 to 10% fewer calories than the Mifflin-St Jeor formula suggests to achieve the same weight maintenance. For Elena, this would reduce her maintenance estimate from 1,928 to approximately 1,735 to 1,830 kcal/day. This is not a cause for despair – it is a reason to use real-world observation (body weight, energy level, blood sugar response) to calibrate the calculation over time rather than treating the initial number as exact.

The Weight Loss Caloric Deficit: How Much Is Safe?

One pound of body fat contains approximately 3,500 kcal of stored energy. A consistent caloric deficit of 500 kcal per day theoretically produces approximately 0.5 kg (1 pound) of weight loss per week. This is the most commonly cited rule in weight management, and it is approximately correct over the first several weeks. Over longer periods, metabolic adaptation reduces the rate of loss – the body partially compensates for caloric restriction by reducing RMR.

For T2DM patients on medications that lower blood sugar, aggressive caloric restriction carries an important safety risk: hypoglycemia. Sulfonylureas and insulin lower blood sugar independently of food intake, meaning that a large caloric deficit combined with these medications can produce dangerously low blood glucose. A deficit of no more than 500 kcal per day is generally safe for most T2DM patients, and any caloric restriction beyond moderate should be discussed with the prescribing physician before implementation.

For Elena's weight loss target (approximately 20 pounds over 10 to 12 months, a rate of approximately 0.5 kg per week):

Target intake = TDEE − 500 kcal = 1,928 − 500 ≈ 1,430 kcal/day

This is Elena's starting weight loss caloric target — to be observed for four weeks and adjusted based on actual results.

Macronutrient Distribution: The Evidence for T2DM

Within the caloric budget, how should Elena distribute her calories among carbohydrates, protein, and fat? This is one of the most contested questions in nutritional science, with proponents of low-fat, low-carbohydrate, very low-carbohydrate (ketogenic), and Mediterranean patterns all presenting supporting evidence.

For T2DM specifically, the current evidence best supports a moderate carbohydrate restriction rather than either extreme. A 2019 systematic review and meta-analysis by Sainsbury and colleagues comparing low-carbohydrate (<130g/day), moderate-carbohydrate (130–225g/day), and high-carbohydrate (>225g/day) diets in T2DM found that low-carbohydrate produced the largest HbA1c reductions at 3 months but that the advantage over moderate carbohydrate was largely lost at 12 months due to lower adherence. The moderate carbohydrate approach produced more durable improvements because it was more sustainable.[49]

The macronutrient distribution with the strongest evidence for both glycemic control and long-term adherence in T2DM:

Carbohydrates: 40 to 45% of calories (predominantly low-GL sources)

Protein: 25 to 30% of calories (1.2 to 1.5g per kg body weight)

Fat: 30 to 35% of calories (predominantly unsaturated, rich in omega-3)

For Elena at 1,430 kcal/day:

Carbohydrates: 1,430 × 0.42 ÷ 4 kcal/g ≈ 150g per day

Protein: 1,430 × 0.27 ÷ 4 kcal/g ≈ 96g per day (1.2g/kg × 80.7 kg = 97g — consistent)

Fat: 1,430 × 0.31 ÷ 9 kcal/g ≈ 49g per day

These are Elena's daily macronutrient targets — a starting framework to be refined by observation.

Your Personal Caloric Calculation

Use this step-by-step template to calculate your own starting caloric target:

TABLE 1: Personal caloric calculation worksheet. Complete with your own measurements. Treat the result as a starting estimate and adjust after four weeks of observation.

Step	Formula	Your Numbers
1. Your weight in kg	Weight in pounds ÷ 2.205	kg
2. Your height in cm	Height in inches × 2.54	cm
3. Your RMR (women)	(10 × kg) + (6.25 × cm) − (5 × age) − 161	kcal/day
3. Your RMR (men)	(10 × kg) + (6.25 × cm) − (5 × age) + 5	kcal/day
4. Activity multiplier	Sedentary 1.2 / Lightly active 1.375 / Moderate 1.55	x
5. Your TDEE	RMR × activity multiplier	kcal/day
6. T2DM adjustment (optional)	TDEE × 0.92 (reduce by 8% for insulin resistance)	kcal/day
7. Weight loss deficit	Subtract 300–500 kcal for gradual weight loss	kcal/day
8. Carbohydrate target	Daily kcal × 0.42 ÷ 4	g/day
9. Protein target	Body weight in kg × 1.2 to 1.5	g/day
10. Fat target	Remaining calories ÷ 9	g/day

Use this 10-step worksheet to calculate your RMR, TDEE, and daily carbohydrate target

Worked example: Elena — 52 years old, 178 lbs, 5ft 4in, lightly active, T2DM

#	Step	Formula	Elena's result	Your numbers
1	Weight in kg	lbs ÷ 2.205	80.7 kg	___ kg
2	Height in cm	inches × 2.54	162.6 cm	___ cm
3	RMR (women)	(10×kg)+(6.25×cm)−(5×age)−161	**1,402 kcal/day**	___ kcal
3	RMR (men)	(10×kg)+(6.25×cm)−(5×age)+5	—	___ kcal
4	Activity factor	Sedentary 1.2 / Light 1.375 / Mod 1.55	**× 1.375**	× ___
5	TDEE	RMR × activity multiplier	1,928 kcal/day	___ kcal
6	T2DM adjustment	TDEE × 0.92	**1,774 kcal/day**	___ kcal
7	Weight loss deficit	Subtract 300-500 kcal	1,374 kcal/day	___ kcal
8	Carbohydrate target	daily kcal × 0.42 ÷ 4	**144 g/day**	___ g/day
9	Protein target	body weight kg × 1.2-1.5	97-121 g/day	___ g/day
10	Fat target	remaining calories ÷ 9	~60 g/day	___ g/day

Elena's targets at a glance

Calories: 1,374 kcal/day   Carbs: 144 g/day   Protein: 97-121 g/day   Fat: ~60 g/day

These numbers are a starting map, not a destination

Implement for 4-6 weeks, observe what happens to body weight and blood glucose, then adjust. Never eat below your RMR — that is your biological floor.

FIGURE 10. The Mifflin-St Jeor worksheet: calculate your personal RMR, TDEE, and macronutrient targets.

WHAT THIS MEANS FOR YOU

THE BOTTOM LINE

Your total daily energy expenditure — the number of calories your body burns in a day — can be estimated using the Mifflin-St Jeor equation multiplied by an activity factor. For weight loss, subtract 300 to 500 kcal from this number. T2DM with insulin resistance slightly reduces effective metabolic rate, so treat the calculation as an overestimate by about 8% and adjust based on four weeks of real-world observation. Never eat below your resting metabolic rate. The calculation is a map; your body's response to it over four weeks is the territory.

FOR YOUR PHYSICIAN

Mifflin-St Jeor equation validation: Mifflin MD et al., *J Am Diet Assoc* 1990;90:1323–1329. Comparison with Harris-Benedict: Frankenfield D et al., *J Am Diet Assoc* 2005;105:775–789.

Low vs moderate vs high carbohydrate in T2DM: Sainsbury E et al., *Diabetes Res Clin Pract* 2018;139:239–252.

Protein requirements in T2DM and insulin resistance: American Diabetes Association Standards 2023, Section 5 (Facilitating Behavior Change). Higher protein target (1.2–1.5g/kg) is supported by evidence for lean mass preservation during weight loss in insulin-resistant patients.

CHAPTER 13

Carbohydrates

Quality, Quantity, and the Index That Matters

If you have T2DM and have attended any nutritional counseling, you have almost certainly been told to count carbohydrates. The advice is correct but incomplete. Counting carbohydrates tells you how much glucose-producing substrate you are consuming. It does not tell you how quickly that glucose will enter your bloodstream, how much of the carbohydrate will be fermented by gut bacteria rather than absorbed, or whether the carbohydrate comes wrapped in fiber and polyphenols that modify both its glycemic impact and its network effects.

This chapter completes the carbohydrate story. Chapter 5 introduced glycemic index and glycemic load; this chapter provides the reference tables you need to apply those concepts, explains carbohydrate counting for medication management, and addresses the specific glycemic impact of alcohol — a topic that is frequently misunderstood by patients on diabetes medications.

THE SCIENCE BEHIND THIS

Net Carbohydrates vs Total Carbohydrates

The carbohydrate number on a nutrition label includes all carbohydrates: digestible starch, sugars, and dietary fiber. For blood sugar management, the relevant number is net carbohydrates — the carbohydrates that are actually digested and absorbed as glucose:

> Net carbohydrates = Total carbohydrates - Dietary fiber - Sugar alcohols (if present)

Dietary fiber does not raise blood sugar (soluble fiber modestly lowers it; insoluble fiber passes through without absorption). Sugar alcohols (sorbitol, xylitol, maltitol, erythritol) are partially absorbed and have variable glycemic effects — erythritol has essentially zero glycemic impact, while maltitol raises blood sugar almost as much as sugar itself. When reading labels, subtract only erythritol fully; subtract other sugar alcohols by 50% as a conservative estimate.

For a food like cooked lentils (100g serving): Total carbohydrates 20g, Dietary fiber 8g, Net carbohydrates 12g.

For the same serving of white rice: Total carbohydrates 28g, Dietary fiber 0.4g, Net carbohydrates 27.6g.

The lentils provide 56% less digestible carbohydrate than the white rice, despite appearing similar on a total carbohydrate comparison.

The Glycemic Load Reference Table

> The glycemic load (GL) of a food serving is calculated as: GL = GI × net carbohydrates (g) ÷ 100.
>
> GL interpretation: Low GL = 1 to 10; Medium GL = 11 to 19; High GL = 20 or above.

A daily diet with total GL below 80 is associated with significantly better glycemic control and lower HbA1c in T2DM patients than a diet with GL above 120 in multiple prospective studies.

TABLE 2: Glycemic load reference table for common foods. *Resistant starch formation from cooling reduces digestible carbohydrate by approximately 50% — values are estimates.

Source: Atkinson FS et al., Diabetes Care 2008 and Birt DF et al., Adv Nutr 2013.

Food	Serving	GI	Net carbs (g)	GL	Classification
Glucose (reference)	50g	100	50	50	High
White bread	1 slice (30g)	75	14	11	Medium
Whole wheat bread	1 slice (30g)	71	12	9	Low
White rice, cooked	150g	73	38	28	High
Brown rice, cooked	150g	66	34	22	High
Basmati rice, cooked	150g	58	32	19	Medium
Cooled/reheated rice	150g	~40	~19*	~8	Low
Oats, rolled, cooked	250g	55	21	12	Medium
Pasta, al dente	150g	45	38	17	Medium
Pasta, overcooked	150g	65	38	25	High
Lentils, cooked	150g	32	18	6	Low
Chickpeas, cooked	150g	28	22	6	Low
Black beans, cooked	150g	30	24	7	Low
Sweet potato, boiled	150g	63	24	15	Medium
White potato, boiled	150g	82	22	18	Medium
White potato, roasted	150g	111	22	24	High
Apple	120g	36	14	5	Low
Banana, ripe	120g	62	23	14	Medium
Banana, unripe	120g	30	21	6	Low
Watermelon	120g	72	6	4	Low
Orange	130g	43	13	6	Low
Corn flakes	30g	93	25	23	High
Bran flakes	30g	74	18	13	Medium

Continues

TABLE 2: Glycemic load reference table for common foods. *Resistant starch formation from cooling reduces digestible carbohydrate by approximately 50% — values are estimates.

Source: Atkinson FS et al., Diabetes Care 2008 and Birt DF et al., Adv Nutr 2013.

Food	Serving	GI	Net carbs (g)	GL	Classification
Steel-cut oats, cooked	250g	42	21	9	Low
Quinoa, cooked	150g	53	31	16	Medium
Barley, cooked	150g	28	31	9	Low
Dark chocolate 70%+	30g	23	10	2	Low
Milk (whole)	250mL	41	11	5	Low
Yogurt, plain	200g	36	8	3	Low
Carrot, raw	80g	35	6	2	Low
Beetroot, cooked	80g	64	8	5	Low

THE SCIENCE BEHIND THIS

Carbohydrate Counting for Medication Management

For patients on insulin, carbohydrate counting is essential for safe dose calculation. The insulin-to-carbohydrate ratio (ICR) – the number of units of rapid-acting insulin needed per 10 grams of carbohydrate – is individualized for each patient and is typically established with physician and diabetes educator guidance.

For patients on sulfonylureas, a simpler version of carbohydrate awareness is adequate: maintaining consistent carbohydrate intake from meal to meal (rather than precise counting) reduces the unpredictability of blood sugar that can cause hypoglycemia with fixed-dose secretagogues.

The practical framework for carbohydrate counting:

One carbohydrate serving = 15 grams of net carbohydrate

Most adults with T2DM: 3 to 4 servings (45 to 60g) per meal, 1 to 2 servings (15 to 30g) per snack

Using the glycemic load framework: target total daily GL below 80 to 100

Alcohol and Blood Sugar: The Delayed Hypoglycemia Problem

Alcohol presents a specific and frequently misunderstood risk for patients with T2DM, particularly those on insulin or sulfonylureas. The mechanism is counterintuitive: alcohol inhibits hepatic gluconeogenesis — the liver's ability to produce glucose from non-carbohydrate precursors — by competing with glucose precursors for hepatic NAD+ (alcohol metabolism requires NAD+, depleting the cofactor needed for gluconeogenesis).

This means that when a T2DM patient on insulin or a sulfonylurea drinks alcohol, the drug continues to lower blood sugar from the carbohydrate side while alcohol simultaneously blocks the liver's compensatory glucose production. The result is delayed hypoglycemia — which can occur 8 to 16 hours after drinking, often during sleep, when the patient is least able to recognize and respond to it.

The practical implications: **(1)** Never drink on an empty stomach — the carbohydrate in the meal partially offsets the gluconeogenesis inhibition. **(2)** Check blood sugar before bed on evenings when you have consumed alcohol, and eat a carbohydrate-containing snack if blood sugar is below 140 mg/dL. **(3)** Inform your physician of your alcohol consumption so that medication dosing can account for it. **(4)** Dry wine and spirits have lower net carbohydrate content than beer and sweet cocktails — but their hypoglycemia risk from gluconeogenesis inhibition is independent of their carbohydrate content.

Reading a Nutrition Label: The Three Numbers That Matter

On a standard nutrition facts label, three numbers determine a food's glycemic impact:

1. **Total Carbohydrate**: the sum of all carbohydrates including fiber and sugar alcohols
2. **Dietary Fiber:** subtract from total carbohydrate to get net carbohydrate
3. **Total Sugars / Added Sugars:** indicates how much of the carbohydrate is rapidly absorbed simple sugar

The number you are most interested in: Total Carbohydrate Dietary Fiber = Net Carbohydrate (the number that actually affects blood sugar).

A food with 25g total carbohydrate and 12g fiber has only 13g of net carbohydrate — a low-glycemic-load food despite its total carbohydrate content. A food with 25g total carbohydrate and 1g fiber has 24g net carbohydrate — potentially high glycemic load depending on serving size.

The serving size on the label is critical: all numbers on the label refer to the declared serving size, which is frequently smaller than the amount most people actually eat. A "serving" of breakfast cereal is typically 30 grams — approximately three-quarters of a standard cup. Most people pour 60 to 90 grams. Reading the label without adjusting for actual serving size produces systematic underestimation of carbohydrate intake.

WHAT THIS MEANS FOR YOU

THE BOTTOM LINE

The carbohydrate number that matters for blood sugar is net carbohydrate — total carbohydrate minus fiber. Glycemic load (GL = GI × net carbs ÷ 100) is the single most useful number for predicting a food's blood sugar impact. A daily GL below 80 to 100 is associated with significantly better HbA1c than a GL above 120. Alcohol causes delayed hypoglycemia in patients on insulin or sulfonylureas by inhibiting the liver's glucose production — a risk that is independent of the carbohydrate content of the drink and occurs most dangerously during sleep.

FOR YOUR PHYSICIAN

Glycemic index and load comprehensive tables: Atkinson FS et al., *Diabetes Care* 2008;31:2281–2283.

Daily GL and HbA1c in T2DM: Barclay AW et al., *Am J Clin Nutr* 2008;87:627–637.

Alcohol and hepatic gluconeogenesis inhibition: Avogaro A et al., *J Clin Endocrinol Metab* 1993;77:1765–1772. Clinical implications for T2DM patients: American Diabetes Association, *Diabetes Care* 2004;27:S65–S66.

CHAPTER 14

Building the Plate

Portions, Preparation, and the Practical Kitchen

The previous thirteen chapters have established a substantial body of nutritional science: which foods suppress which network nodes, how many calories your body needs, and how to evaluate carbohydrates by their glycemic load rather than their total carbohydrate content. Chapter 14 translates all of this into a plate.

Not a theoretical plate. An actual plate — the one you will eat for lunch today, dinner this evening, and breakfast tomorrow morning. A plate that addresses the glycation cascade, suppresses the inflammatory loop, protects the nerve cells, reduces the hexosamine flux, and delivers the polyphenols that activate SIRT1. A plate that takes fifteen minutes to prepare on a Tuesday evening after a long day at work. A plate that does not require specialty ingredients, significant cooking skill, or a dramatic departure from how you currently eat.

This chapter also completes a topic introduced in Chapter 5: the meal sequencing effect. It adds several new practical interventions that are so simple and so evidence-based that omitting them would be a disservice to every reader who has come this far.

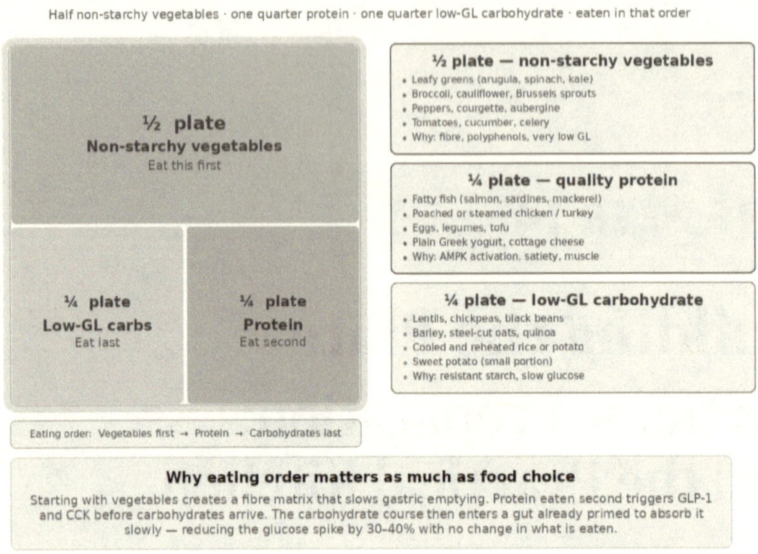

FIGURE 11. The T2DM plate: half non-starchy vegetables, quarter protein, quarter low-GL carbohydrate — eaten in that order.

THE SCIENCE BEHIND THIS

The Network-Optimized Plate

The plate method for T2DM — dividing a standard dinner plate into sections for different food types — has been recommended by diabetes educators for decades. The version presented here updates it with the network biology of Parts I and II:

HALF THE PLATE: Non-starchy vegetables

Not selected merely for their low caloric density and fiber content, but for their specific network-node contributions. Dark leafy greens (spinach, kale, Swiss chard) provide magnesium, lutein, and kaempferol. Broccoli provides sulforaphane precursor and glucoraphanin. Cruciferous vegetables (Brussels sprouts, cauliflower, cabbage) provide indole-3-carbinol and isothiocyanates. Red and yellow peppers provide luteolin and vitamin C. Tomatoes provide lycopene. Purple cabbage and red onion provide quercetin and anthocyanins. Variety within this half-plate is not just nutritional common sense — it is mechanistic diversity.

ONE QUARTER: Protein

Priority: fatty fish (EPA/DHA for PKC suppression, Chapters 6 and 10). Secondary: legumes (quercetin, resistant starch, low GL, prebiotic fiber for the microbiome). Tertiary: poultry (riboflavin, zinc, low saturated fat). Minimize: red and processed meat (high dietary AGE content, arachidonic acid precursor, associated with T2DM progression in epidemiological studies).

ONE QUARTER: Complex carbohydrate

Priority: cooled and reheated grains (resistant starch), legumes (dual protein/carbohydrate), barley (GL ≈ 9, beta-glucan), sweet potato (GL ≈ 15, beta-carotene). Minimize: white refined grains, fresh white rice, overcooked pasta.

Meal Sequencing: The Order of Eating Matters

A series of clinical trials, primarily by Alpana Shukla and colleagues at Cornell's Weill Medical College, has consistently demonstrated that the order in which foods are consumed within a meal significantly affects the postprandial glucose response — even when the total content of the meal is identical.

The mechanism involves gastric emptying rate. When protein and fiber are consumed before carbohydrate, they occupy stomach space, stimulate early cholecystokinin (CCK) and GLP-1 secretion from the gut, slow gastric emptying, and present carbohydrate to the small intestine more slowly. The result is a flattened glucose absorption curve: the same glucose eventually enters the bloodstream, but over a longer period, producing a smaller peak and allowing insulin to keep pace.

In Shukla's 2015 trial, T2DM patients consuming the same meal — chicken, salad, bread, and orange juice — had a 29% lower glucose peak and 37% lower insulin peak at 60 minutes when they ate the protein and salad first and the bread and juice last, compared to eating the bread and juice first. A 2017 follow-up confirmed that the effect was specific to the sequence of the carbohydrate component, not merely to the time elapsed between first and last food.

Vinegar Before Carbohydrate: Dietary Acarbose

Apple cider vinegar, wine vinegar, and other acidic vinegars contain acetic acid at concentrations of 4 to 8%. Acetic acid inhibits alpha-amylase (the enzyme that breaks down complex carbohydrates in the mouth and small intestine) and alpha-glucosidase (the brush border enzyme that releases glucose from disaccharides). These are precisely the enzymes that the prescription drug acarbose inhibits — one of the oldest medications for post-meal blood sugar control.

Multiple RCTs have shown that consuming 1 to 2 tablespoons of vinegar with or before a carbohydrate-containing meal reduces the postprandial glucose spike by 20 to 35%, with a dose-response relationship. The effect is particularly large for refined carbohydrates and smaller for already low-GL foods. A 2004 trial by Johnston and colleagues showed that vinegar consumption before a high-GL meal reduced the 60-minute blood glucose response by 34% compared to control.

The practical application is simple: a small salad dressed with olive oil and wine vinegar before the main course, or a glass of water with one tablespoon of apple cider vinegar 15 minutes before a meal. The acetic acid concentration in the stomach at the time carbohydrates arrive is the relevant variable — timing matters.

The Cooking Method Review and Practical Guide

Chapter 1 established that dry-heat cooking produces dramatically more dietary AGEs than moist-heat cooking. This is the most actionable single cooking habit change for T2DM patients and deserves a practical summary:

MOIST-HEAT METHODS (preferred): Poaching, steaming, slow cooking (crock pot, braising), pressure cooking, microwaving. These methods keep food temperature at or near 100°C and produce minimal AGEs.

DRY-HEAT METHODS (use with modification): Roasting, baking, and sautéing at moderate temperatures (below 180°C) produce moderate AGE levels. Grilling, frying, broiling, and very high-temperature roasting produce the highest AGE levels.

THE ACIDIC MARINADE INTERVENTION: Marinating animal proteins in lemon juice, wine, or vinegar for at least one hour before any dry-heat cooking reduces AGE formation during cooking by approximately 50%. Adding fresh herbs — rosemary, thyme, garlic — to marinades provides additional AGE-inhibiting phenolic compounds.

SPICE ADDITIONS: Cinnamon, cloves, allspice, and ginger contain phenolic compounds that inhibit the Maillard reaction. Adding these spices to high-temperature preparations (roasted sweet potato with cinnamon, grilled meat with a rosemary-garlic marinade) reduces AGE formation modestly.

A Week of Network-Optimized Meals

The following provides one day's meals that integrate every principle in Parts II and III. Each component is annotated with the network node or mechanism it addresses.

TABLE 3: One day of network-optimized meals. Each meal is designed to address multiple network nodes simultaneously while staying within a moderate caloric and glycemic load budget. Total daily GL approximately 57 — comfortably below the target of 80 to 100.

Meal	Components	Network targets addressed	GL
Breakfast	Steel-cut oats (cooled overnight, reheated) with blueberries, ground flaxseed, ground cinnamon, and a tablespoon of walnut pieces. Green tea (no milk).	GCN: resistant starch from cooled oats; POL: quercetin in blueberries; PPP: flaxseed ALA + lignan; HBP: cinnamon insulin sensitization; PKC: walnut ALA; UPR: EGCG from green tea	~14
Mid-morning	30g of broccoli sprouts (raw) with a small handful of capers on the side.	PPP: sulforaphane activating Nrf2; POL: quercetin from capers (70mg+ in 30g)	~2
Lunch	Lentil and red onion soup (with onion skin in cooking liquid) with a tablespoon of extra virgin olive oil drizzled at serving, and a slice of sourdough bread (cold, day-old) with mustard.	GCN: low-GL lentils; POL: quercetin from red onion; NF-κB: oleocanthal from EVOO; PPP: mustard myrosinase activating sulforaphane from any brassica in soup	~18 total
Afternoon snack	A small apple (unpeeled) with 2 tablespoons of almond butter.	GCN: low-GL apple with soluble fiber; NF-κB: vitamin E from almonds; POL: quercetin from apple skin	~7
Dinner	Sequence: Start with green salad dressed with EVOO and wine vinegar. Then: poached salmon with steamed broccoli and turmeric-black pepper cauliflower, with a small serving of barley (cooked the previous day, cooled).	PKC + NF-κB: salmon EPA/DHA; NF-κB: oleocanthal in EVOO; vinegar: alpha-glucosidase inhibition; PPP: broccoli sulforaphane; UPR: curcumin + piperine; HBP: low-GL barley resistant starch	~16 total
Evening supplement	Berberine 500mg with dinner; fish oil 1g EPA+DHA (if fish not at this meal).	HBP: berberine AMPK activation; PKC: additional EPA/DHA	N/A
Daily total GL	150g	~40	~57— well within the target of <80–100

WHAT THIS MEANS FOR YOU

THE BOTTOM LINE

The plate method updated for network biology: half non-starchy vegetables chosen for their specific polyphenol content, one quarter protein prioritizing fatty fish and legumes, one quarter complex carbohydrate choosing cooled grains and legumes for resistant starch. Eat vegetables and protein before carbohydrates – this single sequence change reduces your glucose peak by 30% for the same meal. One tablespoon of vinegar before a high-GL meal inhibits alpha-glucosidase through the same mechanism as acarbose and reduces the glucose spike by 20 to 35%. These interventions are free, require no specialty ingredients, and work every time they are applied.

FOR YOUR PHYSICIAN

Meal sequencing and postprandial glycemia: Shukla AP et al., *Diabetes Care* 2015;38:e98–e99. Follow-up: Shukla AP et al., *BMJ Open Diabetes Res Care* 2017;5:e000440.

Vinegar and alpha-glucosidase inhibition: Johnston CS et al., *Eur J Clin Nutr* 2010;64:1375–1380. Acetic acid as alpha-amylase inhibitor: Leeman M et al., *Eur J Clin Nutr* 2005;59:983–988.

Dietary AGE content by preparation method: Uribarri J et al., *J Am Diet Assoc* 2010;110:911–916.

Red and processed meat in T2DM progression: Pan A et al., *Am J Clin Nutr* 2011;94:1088–1096.

Closing Reflection on Part III

Part III has given you the arithmetic to match the biology of Parts I and II. You now have:

A caloric framework: your personal TDEE calculated from the Mifflin-St Jeor equation, your weight loss target if applicable, and your macronutrient distribution targets for T2DM.

A carbohydrate framework: net carbohydrates as the relevant number, glycemic load as the quality measure, a reference table for your most commonly eaten foods, and a daily GL target below 80 to 100.

A practical kitchen framework: the network-optimized plate, meal sequencing as a free and effortless glucose-spike reducer, vinegar as dietary acarbose, moist-heat cooking as the default method, and the acidic marinade as the modification that makes grilling acceptable.

Part IV now turns from what to eat to when to eat it. The timing of food intake — the spacing between eating windows, the distribution of calories across the day, the fasted state and its molecular consequences — is, as the next three chapters will show, not merely a weight management strategy. It is a direct intervention on the same molecular pathways that medications target. And it is entirely within your control.

Part IV

The Clock as Medicine

When you eat matters as much as what you eat.Intermittent fasting activates the same molecular pathwaysas several diabetes medications. Here is what the evidence shows—and how to do it safely.

The previous three parts have focused on food — its composition, its preparation, its timing within a meal. Part IV steps back from the individual meal and addresses a larger temporal question: not what is on the plate but when the plate is present at all.

The discovery that eating timing matters for metabolic health is not new. Chronobiologists have known for decades that insulin sensitivity, glucose tolerance, and fat oxidation all follow circadian rhythms — rising in the morning and declining through the afternoon. What is new is the mechanistic understanding of why this happens at the cellular level, and the clinical evidence that deliberately manipulating the timing of eating — through intermittent fasting and time-restricted eating — produces metabolic benefits that are only partially explained by caloric restriction.

This part also addresses exercise — not as a weight management strategy but as a direct molecular intervention on the damage network. The AMPK-activating effect of muscular contraction is pharmacologically equivalent to metformin in its immediate cellular consequences. This is not a metaphor. It is a mechanism. Understanding it changes the way you think about a ten-minute walk after dinner.[50, 51]

CHAPTER 15

Why When You Eat Matters as Much as What You Eat

George is fifty-eight years old, works the night shift at a printing company — 11pm to 7am — and has had T2DM for five years. His diet is reasonable by most measures: he cooks at home, avoids junk food, watches his carbohydrate intake. His HbA1c has remained stubbornly at 8.3% despite metformin and a GLP-1 receptor agonist. His endocrinologist is puzzled.

The explanation may lie not in what George eats but in when he eats it. He has his main meals at 1am and 6am — the hours when every metabolic system in his body is, by evolutionary design, expecting him to be asleep. His insulin sensitivity at 1am is approximately 50% of what it would be at 1pm. His melatonin is elevated, suppressing insulin secretion. His liver's glucose production is at its overnight peak. He is eating his largest carbohydrate load at the time when his body is least equipped to handle it.

George is not unusual. He is an extreme version of a pattern that affects millions of people with T2DM who eat late, skip breakfast, or consume most of their calories in the evening. This chapter explains the biology of why this matters — and why shifting calories earlier in the day can produce glycemic improvements without any change in what is consumed.

THE SCIENCE BEHIND THIS

The Circadian Clock: Time-Keeping in Every Cell

Every cell in the human body contains a molecular clock – a self-sustaining oscillator based on a transcription-translation feedback loop involving clock genes (CLOCK, BMAL1, PER1, PER2, CRY1, CRY2). These genes regulate each other's expression in a cycle that repeats approximately every 24 hours. The master clock in the suprachiasmatic nucleus (SCN) of the hypothalamus synchronizes peripheral clocks throughout the body to external time cues – primarily light – through neural and hormonal signals.

The peripheral clocks in the pancreas, liver, skeletal muscle, and adipose tissue regulate the timing of metabolic functions in a tissue-specific manner. In the pancreas, the beta-cell clock controls the timing of insulin secretion – which is highest in the morning and progressively lower in the afternoon and evening. In the liver, the hepatic clock controls gluconeogenesis, glycogen synthesis, and lipid metabolism. In skeletal muscle, the peripheral clock controls GLUT4 expression and insulin-stimulated glucose uptake, which peak in the morning.

The clinical consequence of these rhythms is that glucose tolerance – the ability to process a given glucose load with a given insulin response – is not constant throughout the day. It peaks in the early morning and declines progressively toward the evening. This has been directly demonstrated in controlled studies: the same meal consumed at 8am produces a glucose peak approximately 30 to 40% lower than the same meal consumed at 8pm, even when total caloric intake, physical activity, sleep, and every other variable are held constant. [52]

Melatonin and Insulin: The Evening Suppression

The pineal gland begins secreting melatonin approximately 2 hours before habitual sleep time, reaching peak concentrations in the middle of the night. Melatonin suppresses insulin secretion by binding to MT1 and MT2 receptors on pancreatic beta cells and inhibiting adenylyl cyclase, reducing the cAMP signaling that normally drives insulin secretion. The consequence is reduced insulin availability precisely at the time of night when many people consume their largest meal.[53]

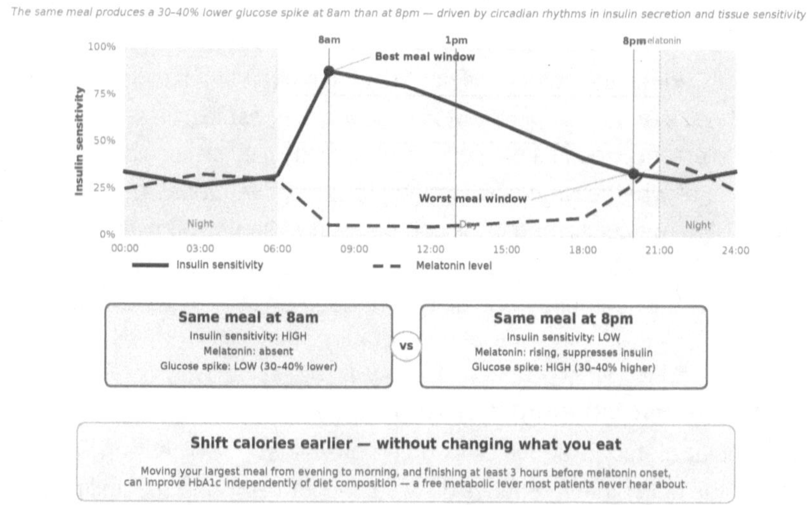

FIGURE 12. Circadian insulin sensitivity: the 24-hour rhythm that determines your glucose response.

This melatonin-insulin interaction helps explain an observation that has puzzled clinicians for decades: why late eating produces disproportionately poor glycemic outcomes even when total caloric intake is matched. It is not simply that the body is less active in the evening – it is that melatonin actively suppresses the insulin secretion needed to handle the carbohydrate load.

A 2022 study in Nature Metabolism showed that individuals who ate their main meal within 1 hour of melatonin onset had significantly higher postprandial glucose and lower insulin secretion than those who ate their main meal at least 3 hours before melatonin onset – even when the meal composition and total caloric intake were identical.[54]

Shift Workers: The Clearest Natural Experiment

Night shift workers provide the most direct human evidence for the metabolic consequences of circadian misalignment – eating and waking at times that are misaligned with the body's internal clock. The epidemiological evidence is striking: night shift workers have a 40% higher prevalence of T2DM than day workers, independent of diet quality, physical activity, BMI, and sleep duration. The metabolic derangement of chronic circadian misalignment includes reduced insulin sensitivity, elevated postprandial glucose, reduced leptin (the satiety hormone), elevated cortisol, and altered gut microbiome composition.[55]

For George, the solution is not to quit his night job. It is to understand that his body's metabolic peak – its window of highest insulin sensitivity and glucose tolerance – occurs during what his circadian clock considers morning, regardless of whether that corresponds to the conventional morning of the solar day. His metabolic morning is approximately 10am to 6pm (after sleeping from roughly 8am to 4pm). Front-loading his calories into this window, eating his largest meal at around noon or 1pm rather than at 1am, would exploit his circadian metabolic peak even within his unconventional sleep schedule.

Why Breakfast Skipping Worsens T2DM

The popular dietary practice of skipping breakfast – which many patients adopt in the belief that it reduces daily caloric intake – has specific negative consequences for T2DM patients that are not simply explained by the caloric redistribution it produces.

A 2015 RCT by Jakubowicz and colleagues showed that T2DM patients who consumed a large breakfast and small dinner had significantly lower HbA1c, postprandial glucose, and insulin requirements than matched patients consuming a small breakfast and large dinner – despite identical total daily caloric intake. The morning-heavy eating pattern exploited the circadian peak of insulin sensitivity; the evening-heavy pattern did not.[56, 57]

In the context of GLP-1 receptor agonists – now among the most commonly prescribed T2DM medications – the circadian argument is particularly compelling. GLP-1 secretion from gut L-cells follows a circadian rhythm peaking in the morning; GLP-1 receptor agonist drugs enhance a signal that is already stronger in the morning. Front-loading calories amplifies the drug's effectiveness rather than working against it.

Time-Restricted Eating vs Intermittent Fasting: Clarifying the Terms

Before Chapter 16 addresses fasting protocols in detail, it is worth clarifying the terminology that is used inconsistently in popular media:

Time-Restricted Eating (TRE): Consuming all calories within a defined eating window each day, without any requirement for caloric restriction within that window. The most studied form is 16:8 (16-hour fasting window, 8-hour eating window). TRE aligns the eating window with the circadian peak of metabolic function — ideally placing the window in the morning to afternoon.

Intermittent Fasting (IF): A broader category encompassing any pattern that involves regular periods of significantly reduced caloric intake. Includes TRE (16:8, 14:10), alternate day fasting (normal eating every other day, severe restriction on alternate days), and the 5:2 protocol (normal eating five days per week, 500 to 600 kcal on two non-consecutive days).

Prolonged fasting: Fasting periods of 24 to 72 hours or more. Requires medical supervision in T2DM patients on glucose-lowering medications.

WHAT THIS MEANS FOR YOU

THE BOTTOM LINE

Insulin sensitivity, glucose tolerance, and the metabolic capacity to handle carbohydrate are not constant throughout the day — they follow a circadian rhythm that peaks in the morning and declines toward the evening. Melatonin, which rises before sleep, actively suppresses insulin secretion. Eating your largest carbohydrate-containing meal in the morning or early afternoon, and finishing your last meal at least 3 hours before sleep, exploits the circadian peak of metabolic function. This produces measurable glycemic improvements even when total caloric intake and food composition are unchanged.

FOR YOUR PHYSICIAN

Circadian clock gene regulation of metabolic function: Bass J, Takahashi JS, *Science* 2010;330:1349–1354. Beta-cell circadian clock: Marcheva B et al., *Nature* 2010; 466:627–631.

Melatonin, MT1/MT2 receptors, and insulin suppression: Rubio-Sastre P et al., *Nat Metab* 2022;4:1508–1519.

Breakfast timing and T2DM outcomes: Jakubowicz D et al., *Diabetes Care* 2015;38:1820–1826.

Shift work and T2DM prevalence: Pan A et al., *PLoS Med* 2011;8:e1001141.

CHAPTER 16

Intermittent Fasting

The Evidence, the Protocols, and the Precautions

Few dietary interventions have generated more public enthusiasm — or more physician caution — than intermittent fasting. The enthusiasm comes from early results: dramatic weight loss, HbA1c improvements, and in some cases apparent remission of T2DM. The caution comes from legitimate concerns about safety in patients on glucose-lowering medications, the quality of existing evidence, and the sustainability of protocols that require periods of significantly restricted or absent eating.

Both the enthusiasm and the caution are justified, and they are not incompatible. Intermittent fasting, applied to the right patient with the right medication adjustments and the right monitoring protocol, is the most powerful non-pharmacological intervention on the hyperglycemic damage network available to a patient with T2DM. Applied to the wrong patient without medication adjustment, it can cause dangerous hypoglycemia.

This chapter presents the evidence for intermittent fasting in T2DM clearly and completely — without the enthusiasm of popular advocates or the reflexive dismissal of clinicians who have not reviewed the mechanistic literature. It then provides step-by-step protocols for the two evidence-based approaches most appropriate for T2DM patients, with the medication safety information that determines whether either is appropriate for you.

THE SCIENCE BEHIND THIS

What Happens in Your Body During a Fast

The fasted state is not merely the absence of the fed state. It is a distinct metabolic condition with specific molecular signatures that are absent when food is continuously available. Understanding these signatures is the mechanistic basis for intermittent fasting's benefits beyond caloric restriction.

Hours 0 to 4 (post-absorptive state): Blood glucose falls toward fasting baseline as the meal's carbohydrates are fully absorbed and processed. Insulin secretion declines. Glucagon begins to rise. Hepatic glycogen begins to be mobilized.

Hours 4 to 12 (early fasting): Hepatic glycogen is the primary glucose source. Insulin is at near-basal levels. The fall in insulin allows AMPK to become more active in liver and muscle — the same kinase that metformin and berberine activate. Fat oxidation begins to increase as insulin's lipogenic suppression of hormone-sensitive lipase is relieved.

Hours 12 to 18 (late fasting): Hepatic glycogen is nearly exhausted. Gluconeogenesis from amino acids and glycerol is the primary glucose source. AMPK is robustly activated. Fat oxidation is now the dominant energy source for muscle and liver. Ketone body production begins — first detectable in blood around 12 to 14 hours of fasting.

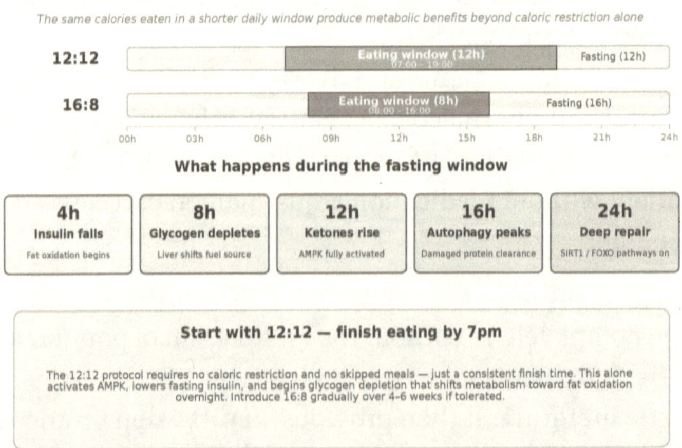

FIGURE 13. Time-restricted eating: 12:12 and 16:8 windows and the metabolic milestones of the fasting state.

Hours 18 to 36 (extended fasting): Ketone bodies become significant energy substrates for the brain, heart, and kidney. Autophagy — cellular self-cleaning through degradation of damaged organelles and misfolded proteins — is substantially upregulated, driven by mTOR inhibition and AMPK activation. Mitochondrial biogenesis begins through PGC-1alpha activation.

AMPK Activation: The Pharmacological Parallel

The AMPK activation that occurs during the late fasting state is pharmacologically equivalent to metformin administration in its cellular consequences. Both metformin and fasting-induced AMPK activation produce: increased glucose uptake in muscle (GLUT4 translocation), reduced hepatic glucose output (inhibition of gluconeogenic enzyme expression), reduced fatty acid synthesis (inhibition of ACC), increased fat oxidation, and activation of SIRT1 (through increased NAD+).

This is not a loose analogy. Foretz and colleagues demonstrated in 2010 that the metabolic effects of metformin are abolished in mice with liver-specific deletion of the AMPK upstream kinase LκB1, confirming that AMPK activation is the primary mechanism of metformin's action. The same AMPK activation produced by 14 to 16 hours of fasting in a human patient is the same molecular event.

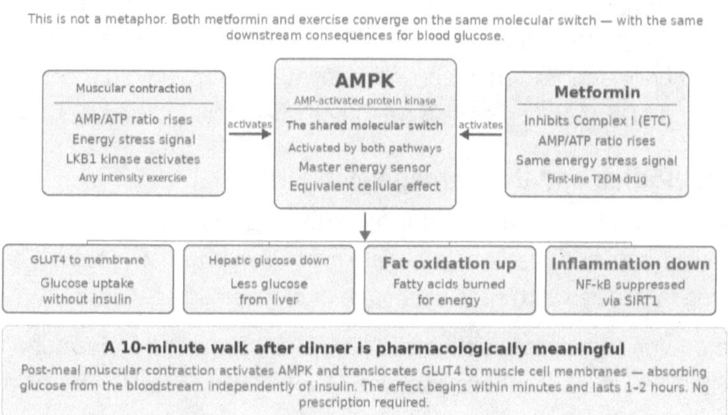

FIGURE 14. Exercise as metformin: muscular contraction and metformin converge on the same AMPK pathway.

The implication is important for T2DM patients on metformin: intermittent fasting and metformin have overlapping mechanisms. Their combination is potentially synergistic — and potentially explains why some patients who add intermittent fasting to metformin therapy achieve HbA1c improvements that exceed what the caloric restriction alone would predict.

Autophagy: The Cellular Cleaning Mechanism

Autophagy — from the Greek for 'self-eating' — is the process by which cells degrade and recycle their own damaged or unnecessary components. Damaged mitochondria, misfolded proteins, protein aggregates, and pathological protein complexes are engulfed in double-membrane vesicles called autophagosomes and delivered to lysosomes for enzymatic degradation. The amino acids, lipids, and other molecules recovered from this process are recycled into new proteins and organelles.

Autophagy is strongly inhibited by the fed state: insulin and amino acids both activate mTOR, which phosphorylates and inactivates the autophagy initiation complex. Fasting removes both of these mTOR activators, allowing autophagy to proceed.

In the context of T2DM, autophagy has specific relevance to the damage network. It degrades the AGE-modified proteins that accumulate in diabetic tissues. It removes dysfunctional mitochondria (mitophagy) that would otherwise amplify the TCA overload described in Chapter 3. It clears the misfolded ER proteins that drive the UPR described in Chapter 11. A 16-hour fasting window, consistently applied, activates autophagy to a degree that meaningful AGE-modified protein clearance is expected to occur.

Ketone Bodies and the Damage Network

The ketone bodies produced during extended fasting — primarily beta-hydroxybutyrate and acetoacetate — are not merely alternative fuels. They are signaling molecules with specific effects on the damage network.

Beta-hydroxybutyrate activates the HCAR2 receptor on immune cells, inhibiting the NLRP3 inflammasome — a key amplifier of NF-κB-driven inflammation. It also serves as a histone deacetylase inhibitor at physiological fasting concentrations, increasing histone acetylation at specific gene promoters in a way that opposes the inflammatory epigenetic reprogramming described in Chapter 4. And it activates PGC-1alpha, the master regulator of mitochondrial biogenesis — the same pathway that the SGLT2 inhibitor mechanism exploits in heart failure.

This means that the ketone bodies produced by 14 to 18 hours of fasting are anti-inflammatory, epigenetically protective, and mitochondrially regenerative — addressing the TCA, NF-κB, and epigenetic nodes of the damage network simultaneously.

CRITICAL MEDICATION SAFETY

Before you fast: the medication safety assessment you must complete.

Medications that require physician review before any fasting protocol:

Sulfonylureas (glipizide, glimepiride, glyburide, glibenclamide): These drugs stimulate insulin secretion regardless of blood glucose. During fasting, when blood glucose is falling, they continue to lower it. Hypoglycemia risk is HIGH. Do not begin any fasting protocol on a sulfonylurea without discussing dose reduction or temporary discontinuation with your physician. Some patients can safely fast on sulfonylureas with dose reduction and increased glucose monitoring; others cannot.

Insulin (all types): Basal insulin must be dose-reduced during fasting periods. Bolus/rapid insulin doses should be eliminated for meals that are skipped. Fasting on standard insulin doses without adjustment causes severe hypoglycemia. Do not fast on insulin without a physician-supervised adjustment protocol.

Meglitinides (repaglinide, nateglinide): Similar mechanism to sulfonylureas. If a meal is skipped, the corresponding dose should be omitted. Discuss with your physician before beginning any fasting protocol.

SGLT2 inhibitors (empagliflozin, dapagliflozin, canagliflozin): Generally safe during 16:8 time-restricted eating. During extended fasting (>24 hours) or very low carbohydrate eating (<50g/day), SGLT2 inhibitors carry a risk of euglycemic diabetic ketoacidosis (DKA) — DKA with normal or near-normal blood glucose, which is easily missed. For extended fasting, most guidelines recommend holding SGLT2 inhibitors. For 16:8 TRE, the risk is low but worth discussing with your physician.

Metformin: Generally safe during 16:8 TRE. Should be taken with food (to reduce gastrointestinal side effects) — take with the first meal of the eating window. During extended fasting (>24 hours), hold metformin in patients at risk for lactic acidosis (eGFR <45, heart failure, liver disease).

GLP-1 receptor agonists (semaglutide, liraglutide, dulaglutide): Generally safe during all fasting protocols. They do not cause hypoglycemia as monotherapy because their insulin-stimulating effect is glucose-dependent. They may increase nausea during the first days of fasting due to their gastroparesis effect — start fasting gradually if on a GLP-1 RA.

DPP-4 inhibitors (sitagliptin, saxagliptin, alogliptin): Generally safe during 16:8 TRE. Low hypoglycemia risk as monotherapy. Take with the first meal of the eating window.

THE CARDINAL RULE: Show this chapter to your physician before beginning any fasting protocol. Bring a list of your medications. Ask specifically about dose adjustments for the protocol you intend to follow. Do not self-adjust insulin doses without physician guidance.

THE SCIENCE BEHIND THIS

The 16:8 Protocol: Evidence in T2DM

The 16:8 protocol — eating within an 8-hour window and fasting for the remaining 16 hours each day — is the most studied and most practically sustainable intermittent fasting approach for T2DM patients. Its evidence base includes:

A 2020 randomized controlled trial by Sutton and colleagues (TREAT trial) in overweight adults with T2DM found that early time-restricted eating (eating window 8am to 2pm) reduced insulin resistance by 3-hour glucose AUC by 18% and reduced blood pressure by 7 mmHg within 5 weeks, with no change in caloric intake between groups. The effect was attributed to circadian alignment rather than caloric restriction.

The most compelling finding across TRE trials is that metabolic improvements occur at caloric intakes that are not significantly different between groups. The timing effect is independent of — and additive to — caloric restriction.

The 5:2 Protocol: Evidence in T2DM

The 5:2 protocol – normal eating on five days per week and severe caloric restriction (500 to 600 kcal) on two non-consecutive days – has its strongest evidence in the DiRECT trial (Diabetes Remission Clinical Trial), conducted in UK primary care settings.

The DiRECT trial used a total diet replacement approach (very low calorie diet of 825 to 853 kcal/day for 12 weeks) rather than the 5:2 protocol specifically, but the weight loss produced (average 10 kg at 12 months) achieved T2DM remission in 46% of participants at 12 months and 36% at 24 months. The remission was primarily mediated by liver fat reduction (reducing hepatic insulin resistance) and partial restoration of beta-cell function.

Subsequent trials using the 5:2 protocol specifically have shown HbA1c reductions of 0.5 to 1.2% compared to standard care, with somewhat lower sustainability than 16:8 TRE at 12 months due to the difficulty of very low calorie days.

How to Start the 16:8 Protocol: A Six-Week Progression

The most common failure mode in starting intermittent fasting is moving too quickly – going from 3 meals plus snacks to a strict 16:8 window in a single day, experiencing hunger, fatigue, and irritability, and abandoning the protocol within a week. A gradual six-week progression produces much higher adherence rates:

Weeks 1 to 2: 12:12. Eat within a 12-hour window (e.g., 7am to 7pm). Stop eating after 7pm. This requires only eliminating late-evening snacking for most people – a change that is manageable and already produces circadian alignment benefits.

Weeks 3 to 4: 14:10. Shift to a 10-hour eating window (e.g., 8am to 6pm). Most people achieve this by delaying breakfast by one hour and moving dinner one hour earlier.

Weeks 5 to 6: 16:8. The full protocol – 8-hour eating window (e.g., 8am to 4pm or 10am to 6pm). The window should be placed in the morning to early afternoon to align with the circadian metabolic peak.

During all stages: drink water, black coffee, or plain tea freely during the fasting window. These beverages do not break the fast's metabolic benefits (they do not stimulate insulin or mTOR) and substantially reduce the hunger that limits adherence in the early weeks.

TABLE 4: Intermittent fasting protocols for T2DM. Medication safety column refers to the specific protocol in isolation; all protocols require physician review of current medications before initiation.

Protocol	Eating window	Fasting window	HbA1c evidence(g)	Best for	Medication safety
12:12 (transitional)	12 hours	12 hours	Modest improvement; primarily circadian alignment benefit	Starting point for all patients; night shift workers aligning window to their metabolic morning	Safe for all T2DM medications with standard precautions
16:8 TRE	8 hours	16 hours	0.5–0.9% HbA1c reduction vs control; 14–36% remission in selected trials	Most T2DM patients; achievable long-term; strongest evidence base	Review required for SU, insulin, meglitinides; generally safe for metformin, GLP-1 RA, DPP4i, SGLT2i
5:2	5 normal days, 2 restricted (500–600 kcal)	2 days severely restricted	0.5–1.2% HbA1c reduction; high remission in significant weight loss context	Patients willing to tolerate 2 very restricted days per week; strongest evidence for T2DM remission	High hypoglycemia risk on SU/ insulin on restricted days — requires dose adjustment or omission
Alternate Day Fasting	Every other day normal, alternating with 25% calorie days	Every other day	Limited T2DM-specific data; effective for weight loss	Not generally recommended as first approach for T2DM due to medication complexity	High complexity for medication management; requires close physician supervision

WHAT THIS MEANS FOR YOU

THE BOTTOM LINE

Intermittent fasting activates AMPK through the same mechanism as metformin, initiates autophagy that clears AGE-modified proteins and dysfunctional mitochondria, and produces ketone bodies that suppress NF-κB inflammation and activate mitochondrial biogenesis. These are not effects of caloric restriction — they are specific to the fasted state. The 16:8 protocol (8-hour eating window) reduces HbA1c by 0.5 to 0.9% beyond dietary changes alone and achieves remission in 14 to 36% of selected T2DM patients. Medication safety review is mandatory before beginning: sulfonylureas and insulin require dose adjustment; SGLT2 inhibitors carry DKA risk during extended fasting.

FOR YOUR PHYSICIAN

TREAT trial (early TRE in T2DM): Sutton EF et al., *Cell Metab* 2018;27:1212–1221.

DiRECT trial: Lean ME et al., *Lancet* 2018;391:541–551. 24-month outcomes: Lean ME et al., *Lancet Diabetes Endocrinol* 2019;7:344–355.

AMPK as primary metformin mechanism: Foretz M et al., *J Clin Invest* 2010;120:2355–2369.

Beta-hydroxybutyrate and NLRP3 inflammasome: Youm YH et al., *Nat Med* 2015;21:263–269. BHB as histone deacetylase inhibitor: Shimazu T et al., *Science* 2013;339:211–214.

Euglycemic DKA with SGLT2 inhibitors: Fadini GP et al., *BMJ* 2017;356:i6979.

CHAPTER 17

Exercise as Network Medicine

The instruction to exercise is among the most frequently given and least specifically justified pieces of medical advice in T2DM management. Patients are told that exercise improves blood sugar control, helps with weight loss, and reduces cardiovascular risk. All of this is true. But none of it explains the mechanism precisely enough to make the instruction feel urgent and specific rather than vague and optional.

This chapter explains the mechanism. The molecular events that occur in a skeletal muscle cell during a ten-minute brisk walk are as specific, as documented, and as relevant to the hyperglycemic damage network as the mechanism of any drug in your medication cabinet. Understanding those events changes the way you think about physical activity — not as a lifestyle recommendation appended to the real treatment, but as a pharmacological intervention that operates through mechanisms that no drug currently replicates.

THE SCIENCE BEHIND THIS

AMPK Activation by Muscular Contraction: Exercise as Pharmacology

When a skeletal muscle cell contracts, it consumes ATP – the cell's energy currency. As ATP is consumed, AMP accumulates (ATP → ADP → AMP). The rising AMP/ATP ratio activates AMPK, the master energy sensor described throughout this book as the shared mechanism of metformin, berberine, and the fasting state.

Exercise-induced AMPK activation in muscle produces a specific and immediately clinically relevant effect: translocation of GLUT4 glucose transporters to the cell surface. GLUT4 is the insulin-responsive glucose transporter — under resting conditions, GLUT4 is held in intracellular storage vesicles and only translocates to the cell membrane when insulin binds its receptor and activates the PI3K-Akt signaling cascade. During exercise, AMPK provides a completely independent, insulin-independent signal for GLUT4 translocation.

The consequence is extraordinary: skeletal muscle takes up glucose from the bloodstream during and immediately after exercise without any insulin. A ten-minute walk after a meal activates AMPK in the large muscle groups of the legs, translocates GLUT4 to the muscle cell surface, and drives glucose from the postprandial glucose peak directly into muscle without waiting for the insulin response. The postprandial glucose spike is blunted by approximately 25 to 30% from a ten-minute post-meal walk — before a single unit of insulin has acted.

For patients with impaired insulin secretion or insulin resistance, this insulin-independent mechanism is particularly valuable. It represents a route to glucose disposal that does not depend on the compromised insulin signaling pathway.

The Post-Meal Walk: The Minimum Effective Dose

The clinical evidence for post-meal walking as a glucose-lowering intervention is some of the most practical in the exercise literature. A 2013 study by DiPietro and colleagues compared 15-minute walks after each meal versus a single 45-minute walk at a fixed time of day in older adults with impaired glucose regulation. The post-meal walk group had significantly better 24-hour glucose profiles than the single-walk group, with the largest improvement in the afternoon and evening periods — precisely when circadian insulin sensitivity is declining.

A 2016 meta-analysis of post-meal exercise in T2DM confirmed that walking for 10 to 15 minutes after meals reduces postprandial glucose by 12 to 22 mg/dL compared to sitting after meals — a reduction comparable to a low-dose sulfonylurea, achieved by walking.

The timing sensitivity is important: the glucose-lowering benefit of a post-meal walk is most pronounced when the walk occurs within 30 to 60 minutes of the meal, when the postprandial glucose peak is occurring. Walking 2 hours after a meal, when glucose has already partially returned to baseline, produces a smaller effect.

Resistance Training: The Metabolic Sink

Resistance training — working muscles against load, whether through weights, resistance bands, bodyweight exercises, or any other form — produces benefits for T2DM patients that go beyond the immediate glucose-lowering of aerobic exercise. Its most important metabolic effect is the long-term one: the building or preservation of muscle mass.

Skeletal muscle is the largest glucose-consuming tissue in the body, accounting for 70 to 80% of insulin-stimulated glucose uptake under euglycemic clamp conditions. More muscle mass means a larger metabolic sink — more tissue available to absorb glucose from the bloodstream in response to insulin. A 5% increase in skeletal muscle mass produces approximately a 20 to 35% improvement in whole-body insulin sensitivity, an effect that persists for 24 to 48 hours after each resistance training session.

This duration of effect is mechanistically important. Resistance training activates AMPK during the session, producing the acute GLUT4 translocation benefit. It also activates mTOR (through a different pathway than the mTOR inhibition of fasting) to stimulate muscle protein synthesis, rebuilding and enlarging the muscle fibers. The enlarged muscle fibers contain more GLUT4, more mitochondria, and more insulin receptor — the improved insulin sensitivity that persists between sessions.

High-Intensity Interval Training (HIIT) in T2DM

HIIT — brief periods of high-intensity effort alternating with recovery periods — produces greater improvements in HbA1c, insulin sensitivity, and VO2max per unit of time than moderate continuous exercise in multiple RCTs in T2DM patients. The mechanism involves greater AMPK activation (because high-intensity work creates larger ATP deficits), greater mitochondrial biogenesis through PGC-1alpha, and more extensive GLUT4 upregulation than moderate exercise.

The most studied and most accessible HIIT protocol for T2DM patients is the "1-minute hard, 1-minute easy" interval: 10 rounds of 1 minute at high effort alternating with 1 minute of easy walking, for a total of 20 minutes including warmup and cooldown. Borg scale effort during the high-intensity intervals should be 7 to 8 out of 10 — hard enough to prevent holding a conversation, not so hard as to be unsustainable for 1 minute.

A 2014 RCT by Little and colleagues showed that 3 sessions per week of 10 one-minute high-intensity intervals reduced HbA1c by 0.5% more than moderate continuous exercise matched for total exercise time over 12 weeks. The time investment was 30 minutes per session, 3 sessions per week — 90 minutes total per week of active exercise time.

Exercise and the Damage Network: The Node-by-Node View

Acute exercise: AMPK activation reduces TCA cycle overload (by increasing mitochondrial efficiency and reducing superoxide production), reduces hexosamine pathway flux (by lowering glucose availability), and activates SIRT1 (through AMPK-NAD+ elevation). Post-exercise GLUT4 translocation reduces postprandial glucose exposure and therefore GCN node activation.

Chronic exercise: Mitochondrial biogenesis through PGC-1alpha reduces the mitochondrial superoxide production that is the central amplifier of all four classical damage pathways. Muscle mass increase reduces insulin resistance and hexosamine pathway activity. Exercise-induced adipose tissue mobilization reduces the ectopic fat that activates PKC in hepatocytes and cardiac myocytes.

The anti-inflammatory effect of regular aerobic exercise — mediated through reduction of visceral adipose tissue, IL-6 secretion from muscle (which paradoxically has anti-inflammatory effects when produced during exercise), and reduced NF-κB activation — addresses the NF-κB inflammatory convergence node through a mechanism entirely independent of dietary polyphenol interventions. Exercise and the dietary anti-inflammatory strategy of Chapter 6 are complementary, not redundant.

TABLE 5: Exercise types, doses, and evidence for T2DM. All evidence is for T2DM patients specifically. HbA1c effects are relative to non-exercising controls on equivalent diet and medication.

Exercise type	Minimum dose	Immediate glucose effect	Sustained metabolic effect	Primary network node addressed	Evidence in T2DM
Post-meal walk	10–15 minutes within 30–60 min of meal	12–22 mg/dL reduction in postprandial glucose peak	Modest if single session; cumulative if daily	GCN: reduces postprandial glucose exposure; HBP: reduces hexosamine flux	Strong RCT evidence; DiPietro 2013, multiple meta-analyses
Moderate aerobic (brisk walking, cycling)	150 min/week (30 min × 5)	Modest acute glucose lowering during and 24–48h post	Improved VO2max, reduced HbA1c 0.5–0.7%	TCA: mitochondrial efficiency; NF-κB: reduced inflammatory adipokines	ADA guideline-endorsed; large body of RCT evidence
Resistance training	2–3 sessions/week, 8–10 exercises, 2–3 sets each	Moderate acute glucose lowering	Improved insulin sensitivity 24–48h per session; long-term: increased muscle mass = improved metabolic sink	HBP: reduced insulin resistance; TCA: increased mitochondrial density	Strong RCT evidence; additional HbA1c reduction 0.3–0.5% beyond aerobic alone
HIIT (10×1 min high, 1 min easy)	3 sessions/week, 20 min total	Strong acute glucose lowering; AMPK activation greater than moderate exercise	Superior HbA1c reduction per time unit vs moderate exercise; greater mitochondrial biogenesis	All nodes: maximum AMPK activation; strongest PGC-1alpha response	Little JA et al. 2014; multiple RCTs showing superiority per unit time
Combined (aerobic + resistance)	150 min aerobic + 2–3 resistance sessions/week	Additive to individual modes	Greatest HbA1c reduction of any exercise regimen: 0.9–1.1% beyond diet alone	Broadest node coverage	Sigal RJ et al. NEJM 2007: combined superior to either alone

WHAT THIS MEANS FOR YOU

THE BOTTOM LINE

Skeletal muscle contraction activates AMPK through the same molecular mechanism as metformin — rising AMP/ATP ratio — and drives GLUT4 glucose transporters to the cell surface independent of insulin. A ten-minute walk within 60 minutes of a meal lowers the postprandial glucose peak by 12 to 22 mg/dL through this mechanism. Resistance training builds the muscle mass that is your body's largest glucose-consuming organ, improving insulin sensitivity for 24 to 48 hours after every session. HIIT produces the greatest HbA1c improvement per unit of time. Combined aerobic plus resistance training produces HbA1c reductions of 0.9 to 1.1% beyond diet alone — equivalent to a second medication.

FOR YOUR PHYSICIAN

AMPK activation by muscle contraction and GLUT4 translocation: Richter EA, Hargreaves M, *Physiol Rev* 2013;93:993–1017.

Post-meal walking: DiPietro L et al., *Diabetes Care* 2013;36:3262–3268. Meta-analysis: Buffet-Batillon S et al., *Diabetes Metab* 2018;44:295–303.

Combined aerobic + resistance training in T2DM: Sigal RJ et al., *Ann Intern Med* 2007; 147:357–369.

HIIT vs moderate continuous exercise in T2DM: Little JP et al., *J Appl Physiol* 2014;116:1274–1282.

Exercise and mitochondrial biogenesis via PGC-1alpha: Holloszy JO, *J Appl Physiol* 2011;110:1234–1235.

Closing Reflection on Part IV

Part IV has made an argument that most dietary books do not make: that the timing of eating and the act of physical movement are pharmacological interventions in the same sense that a tablet or injection is pharmacological — because they activate the same molecular pathways, at the same molecular targets, through mechanisms that are as precisely documented as any drug's mechanism of action.

> The ten-minute post-meal walk activates GLUT4 translocation through AMPK — the same kinase that metformin activates. The 16-hour fast activates autophagy that clears AGE-modified proteins — a cellular cleansing that no current medication performs. The ketone bodies of the fasted state inhibit the NLRP3 inflammasome and oppose the inflammatory epigenetic marks of the damage network. These are not vague lifestyle benefits. They are specific molecular interventions.
>
> What makes Part IV's interventions uniquely powerful is that they are entirely within your control at zero cost — no prescription, no pharmacy visit, no insurance coverage required. The walk after dinner is free. The decision to stop eating at 7pm is free. The AMPK activation that results is identical regardless of whether it was triggered by metformin or by thirty minutes of exercise.

Part V now turns to the most novel science in the book: the polyphenols that address the damage network at the molecular level, and the bitter receptor discovery that is revealing an entirely new dimension of how food talks to the gut.

Part V

Polyphenols, Supplements, and the Bitter Frontier

The most novel section of the book.Plant compounds that directly suppress the damage network.The bitter receptor discovery that is rewriting our understandingof how food talks to the gut.

Part V enters territory that most dietary books for diabetes patients do not visit: the pharmacology of plant compounds at the molecular level, and a discovery published between 2008 and 2024 that is fundamentally changing our understanding of how the gut processes food signals and communicates with the rest of the body.

The polyphenols described in this part are not vitamins. They are not essential nutrients whose absence causes deficiency diseases. They are pharmacologically active compounds that plants produce for their own biological purposes — defense against pathogens, UV radiation, and herbivores — and that happen to interact with the same molecular targets that diabetes drugs target, through mechanisms that are now understood in sufficient detail to justify their use as deliberate therapeutic tools.

The bitter receptor story in Chapter 20 is the most scientifically novel content in this book. It describes a family of receptors discovered in the gut in the early 2000s — receptors that were originally thought to exist only on the tongue — whose activation by bitter food compounds triggers GLP-1 secretion through a mechanism structurally analogous to what semaglutide and liraglutide do pharmacologically. If you have been prescribed a GLP-1 receptor agonist, or if your physician has discussed one, this chapter will change the way you think about the bitter foods you may have spent a lifetime avoiding.

CHAPTER 18

What Polyphenols Actually Do

Walk into any health food store and you will find shelves of supplements labeled "rich in antioxidants," "high in polyphenols," "packed with phytonutrients." These claims are not false — polyphenol-rich foods and supplements do contain biologically active compounds. But the framing reduces something pharmacologically complex to a marketing category, and the marketing category obscures the actual mechanism.

Polyphenols are not antioxidants in the way that a bucket of water is a fire suppressor — by simply absorbing reactive oxygen species and being consumed in the process. At physiological concentrations in tissue, polyphenols act primarily as *signaling molecules:* they activate enzymes, inhibit enzymes, modify gene expression, and alter the function of transcription factors. Their antioxidant effect, to the extent that it is relevant, is largely indirect — through upregulation of the cell's own enzymatic antioxidant systems, not through direct chemical neutralization of free radicals. This distinction changes everything about how to use them.

THE SCIENCE BEHIND THIS

The Xenohormesis Hypothesis: Why Plants Make Your Medicine

Plants under environmental stress – drought, UV exposure, pathogen attack, soil nutrient scarcity – produce higher concentrations of polyphenols and other secondary metabolites. The evolutionary logic from the plant's perspective is clear: these compounds protect against UV damage, deter herbivores, and inhibit competing microorganisms. From the perspective of animals that eat stressed plants, something interesting follows.

In 2008, David Sinclair and Konrad Lichten proposed the xenohormesis hypothesis: that animals have evolved to detect the chemical stress signals in the plants they eat and to use those signals as advance warning of environmental adversity. A plant producing stress polyphenols is signaling that conditions are deteriorating. An animal consuming that plant activates its own stress-resistance pathways — AMPK, SIRT1, Nrf2, autophagy — in preparation for the adversity ahead.[58]

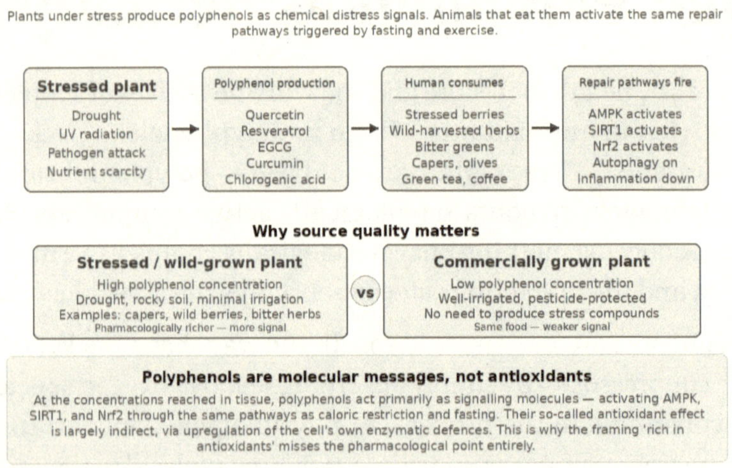

FIGURE 15. Xenohormesis: stressed plants produce polyphenols that activate human repair pathways.

The clinical implication is that polyphenols from stressed plants are essentially molecular messages that say: times are hard, conserve energy, activate repair mechanisms, reduce inflammation, clear damaged proteins. These are precisely the same metabolic programs that caloric restriction, fasting, and exercise activate. Polyphenols are, in this framework, chemical mimics of the fasting signal — which is why their effects so closely parallel those of dietary restriction.

This also explains why organically grown, pesticide-free, and drought-stressed plants often have higher polyphenol content than conventionally grown, well-irrigated counterparts. The conventionally grown plant has no reason to produce stress compounds. The stressed plant produces them abundantly. This is not an argument for abandoning food safety standards — it is an explanation for why wild-harvested berries, capers from rocky Mediterranean hillsides, and bitter greens from nutrient-poor soils are pharmacologically richer than their commercially cultivated equivalents.

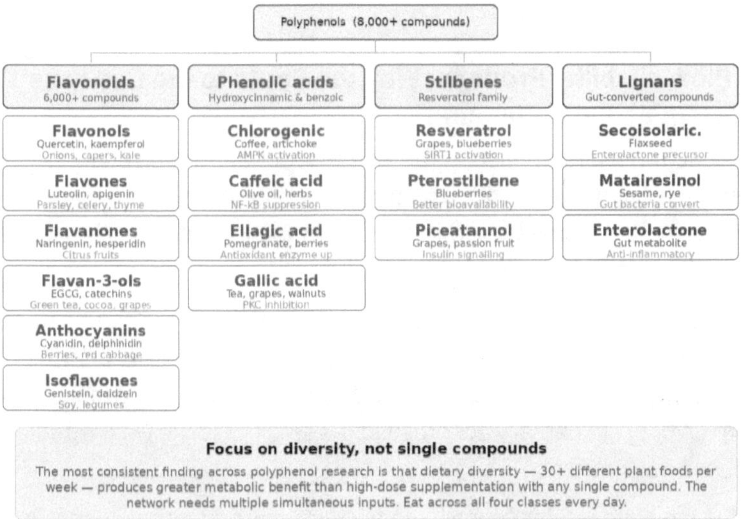

FIGURE 16. Polyphenol class taxonomy: four major classes, subclasses, and key dietary examples.

Polyphenol Classes: A Brief Taxonomy

Over 8,000 polyphenolic compounds have been identified in plants. They are organized into several major classes:[59]

Flavonoids (largest class, over 6,000 compounds): Includes flavonols (quercetin, kaempferol), flavones (luteolin, apigenin), flavanones (naringenin from citrus), isoflavones (genistein, daidzein from soy), flavan-3-ols (catechins from tea, procyanidins from grapes and cocoa), and anthocyanins (the blue-red pigments from berries, red cabbage, and red onion).

Phenolic acids: Includes hydroxycinnamic acids (caffeic acid, chlorogenic acid from coffee and artichoke) and hydroxybenzoic acids (gallic acid, ellagic acid from pomegranate).

Stilbenes: Resveratrol and its relatives from grapes, blueberries, and Japanese knotweed.

Lignans: Secoisolariciresinol from flaxseed, enterolactone (a lignan metabolite produced by gut bacteria).

Tannins: Condensed tannins (proanthocyanidins from grapes, apples, cinnamon) and hydrolysable tannins (ellagitannins from pomegranate, walnuts).

The Bioavailability Problem: Why the Route to the Cell Is as Important as the Compound

The most important and least appreciated fact about polyphenols is their variable and often low oral bioavailability. Most polyphenols are not absorbed as the compounds measured in food composition tables. They undergo substantial modification during digestion:

In the mouth and stomach: Acid hydrolysis cleaves sugar groups from polyphenol glycosides, releasing the aglycone form. Salivary enzymes begin polyphenol metabolism. Some compounds (like quercetin glucoside from onions) are partially absorbed in the small intestine via the sodium-glucose transporter.

In the small intestine: Phase II metabolism in the intestinal epithelium converts polyphenols to sulfate and glucuronide conjugates, reducing absorption of the intact compound. This is particularly problematic for curcumin (less than 1% bioavailability) and resveratrol (rapidly conjugated to sulfate and glucuronide).

In the colon: The microbiome transforms polyphenol glycosides and polymers into smaller phenolic metabolites — urolithins from ellagitannins, equol from soy isoflavones, enterolactone from flaxseed lignans — that are sometimes more bioactive than the parent compound and are absorbed into the circulation from the colon.[60]

The consequences for how to use polyphenols: (1) Whole food sources generally outperform isolated supplements for the same nominal polyphenol content because the food matrix modifies absorption favorably. (2) The gut microbiome composition determines polyphenol metabolism — individual responses to the same polyphenol source vary substantially based on microbial community. (3) Lipophilic formulations, piperine co-administration, and micronization can dramatically improve bioavailability of specific compounds. (4) The most relevant question is not how much polyphenol is in the food but how much bioavailable polyphenol reaches the target tissue.

Primary vs Secondary Mechanisms: Signaling Over Scavenging

At tissue concentrations achieved from food consumption, polyphenols are too dilute to act as significant chemical antioxidants — the concentration of reactive oxygen species in a cell during oxidative stress far exceeds the concentration of polyphenol metabolites at those same concentrations. What polyphenols do at physiological concentrations is modulate signaling pathways:[61]

Enzyme inhibition: Quercetin inhibits aldose reductase, as described in Chapter 8. Curcumin inhibits IKK-beta, blocking NF-κB activation. EGCG inhibits IRE1-alpha, reducing ER stress signaling. These are direct enzyme-compound interactions.

Transcription factor activation: Sulforaphane activates Nrf2. Resveratrol activates SIRT1. Berberine activates AMPK upstream of multiple transcription factor pathways. These are effects that cascade through hundreds of downstream gene products.

Receptor modulation: Isoflavones bind estrogen receptors. EGCG binds the 67-kDa laminin receptor and modulates its downstream signaling. Bitter polyphenols activate TAS2R bitter taste receptors — the subject of Chapter 20.

WHAT THIS MEANS FOR YOU

THE BOTTOM LINE

Polyphenols are not antioxidants in the bucket-of-water sense. They are signaling molecules that activate and inhibit specific enzymes and transcription factors at concentrations achievable through diet. Their bioavailability is variable and often low — modified by digestion, conjugation in the gut wall, and microbial transformation in the colon. Understanding this changes how you choose and use them: whole food sources, fat-containing preparations, and a healthy microbiome are all part of the delivery system, not just the molecule itself.FOR

FOR YOUR PHYSICIAN

Xenohormesis hypothesis: Howitz KT, Sinclair DA, *Cell* 2008;133:387–391.

Polyphenol bioavailability and gut microbiome transformation: Manach C et al., *Am J Clin Nutr* 2004;79:727–747. Urolithin production from ellagitannins: Selma MV et al., *J Agric Food Chem* 2009;57:7254–7263.

Polyphenol signaling vs antioxidant mechanisms: Forman HJ et al., *Arch Biochem Biophys* 2014;559:100–110.

CHAPTER 19

The Star Polyphenols

Evidence and Practical Guide

Chapter 18 established the conceptual framework: polyphenols are signaling molecules with specific molecular targets, variable bioavailability, and effects that depend on microbiome composition. This chapter applies that framework to the five polyphenols with the most robust clinical evidence in T2DM and metabolic disease: berberine, resveratrol, curcumin, EGCG, and quercetin. Each is assessed by its mechanism, the strength of its clinical evidence, the practical considerations for its use, and its drug interaction profile.

For use alongside dietary changes. Always discuss with your physician before starting any supplement.

Supplement	Dose	When to take	Nodes targeted	Evidence level
Berberine	500 mg × 3/day	With meals	GCN · HBP · PKC	Strong — multiple RCTs
Magnesium glycinate	300–400 mg/day	Evening	GCN · HBP	Strong — cofactor deficiency
Omega-3 EPA/DHA	2–4 g/day	With largest meal	PKC · NF-kB	Strong — multiple RCTs
Curcumin + piperine	500 mg + 5 mg	With fat-containing meal	UPR · NF-kB	Moderate — bioavailability key
Alpha-lipoic acid	300–600 mg/day	Before meals	PPP · POL	Moderate — neuropathy focus
Vitamin D3 + K2	2,000–4,000 IU	With fat meal	NF-kB · UPR	Moderate — if deficient
Zinc	15–25 mg/day	With food	GCN · POL	Moderate — T2DM depletion
Chromium picolinate	200–400 mcg/day	With meals	HBP · GCN	Modest — insulin sensitivity

With meals	**Before meals**	**With fat meal**	**Evening**
Take with first bite of meal	30 min before — pre-meal window	Fat-soluble: needs dietary fat	Overnight circadian tissue repair

Lead with diet — use supplements to amplify

The evidence hierarchy places berberine and omega-3 at the top, with strong RCT support across multiple endpoints. Start with these two before adding others. Introduce one supplement at a time over 4-week intervals to identify any effects clearly. Supplements amplify a good diet — they cannot rescue a poor one.

FIGURE 17. Evidence-based supplement guide: dose, timing, network targets, and evidence level.

These five were introduced in earlier chapters in the context of specific network nodes. This chapter provides the complete picture for each — the full evidence base, the dose, the formulation, and the specific patient situations where the evidence is strongest. Consider this chapter your reference for the polyphenol supplement decisions you may be considering.

THE SCIENCE BEHIND THIS

Berberine: The Most Evidence-Based Dietary Supplement for T2DM

Berberine's complete evidence profile in T2DM is the strongest of any dietary supplement in this chapter, with 14 randomized controlled trials, a consistent effect size, and direct mechanistic alignment with approved pharmacotherapy.

Mechanism: Inhibition of mitochondrial Complex I → increased AMP/ATP ratio → AMPK activation → reduced hepatic gluconeogenesis, increased muscle glucose uptake, improved insulin sensitivity, reduced hexosamine pathway flux, SIRT1 activation. Secondary mechanisms include gut TAS2R bitter receptor activation (Chapter 20), microbiome modulation toward Akkermansia and Bifidobacterium, and NF-κB suppression.

Evidence: The landmark 2008 Yin trial (n=116) showed berberine 500mg three times daily achieved HbA1c reduction of 2.0% from baseline vs 1.9% for metformin – non-inferior in head-to-head comparison. A subsequent 2012 meta-analysis of 14 RCTs (n=1,068) showed consistent HbA1c reduction of 0.9 to 1.2% vs placebo, with additional significant effects on fasting glucose, postprandial glucose, and triglycerides.[62]

A 2015 Cochrane-methodology systematic review concluded that berberine combined with lifestyle intervention was superior to lifestyle intervention alone, and berberine plus oral hypoglycemic agents was superior to oral hypoglycemics alone, for HbA1c reduction. No equivalent systematic review evidence exists for any other polyphenol supplement in T2DM.[63]

Dose: 500mg three times daily with meals. The with-meals requirement is important: bile secretion stimulated by food significantly improves berberine absorption. Some clinical trials use 300mg three times daily as a starting dose.

Formulation: Standard berberine hydrochloride is the most studied form. Berberine phytosome (berberine complexed with phosphatidylcholine) and dihydroberberine (a more bioavailable reduced form) are available and may offer equivalent or superior effects at lower doses.

Drug interactions: Inhibits CYP2D6 (relevant for metoprolol, paroxetine, codeine) and CYP3A4 (relevant for statins, cyclosporine, some calcium channel blockers). Produces additive glucose lowering with metformin, insulin, and sulfonylureas – monitor blood glucose when adding berberine to existing therapy. Inhibits P-glycoprotein – may increase absorption of drugs that are P-gp substrates.

Resveratrol: The SIRT1 Activator

Resveratrol's story is complicated by controversy about its primary mechanism and by disappointing clinical trial results at the food-achievable doses. The initial enthusiasm following Howitz and Sinclair's 2003 discovery of resveratrol as a SIRT1 activator has been tempered by subsequent evidence that resveratrol's SIRT1 activation may be indirect (through increased NAD+ levels) rather than direct allosteric activation. Despite this mechanistic revision, the downstream metabolic effects of resveratrol – AMPK activation, reduced inflammatory cytokines, improved insulin sensitivity – are well-documented and consistent across multiple cell types and animal models.[64]

In humans with T2DM, the evidence is mixed. A 2012 RCT by Bhatt and colleagues showed that resveratrol 250mg per day for 3 months reduced HbA1c by 0.5%, fasting glucose by 26 mg/dL, and systolic blood pressure by 4.5 mmHg in T2DM patients on standard medication. Several subsequent trials showed similar modest effects; others showed no effect. The heterogeneity is largely explained by the bioavailability problem: standard resveratrol is rapidly conjugated to sulfate and glucuronide in the intestinal wall and achieves low free plasma concentrations.

Dose: 150 to 500mg per day of micronized resveratrol or resveratrol with piperine (to inhibit glucuronidation, as with curcumin). Standard resveratrol powder at these doses is likely to have minimal effect.

Food sources: Trans-resveratrol content (the bioactive form) per 100g: Japanese knotweed root (40,000 to 110,000 mcg – by far the highest source, used in supplements), red wine (64 to 640 mcg per 100mL – insufficient for pharmacological effect), blueberries (8 to 47 mcg), dark grapes (4 to 32 mcg). Food sources are insufficient to produce the tissue concentrations associated with clinical benefit.

Best indication: Patients specifically concerned about SIRT1 activation and epigenetic memory (Chapter 4), NASH (Chapter 11's hepatic ER stress context), and neuropathy protection (polyol pathway node, Chapter 8).

Curcumin: The Multi-Node Suppressor

Curcumin has the broadest network coverage of any single polyphenol: IKK-beta inhibition (NF-κB, Chapter 6), Nrf2 activation (antioxidant defense, Chapter 7), IRE1-alpha inhibition (ER stress, Chapter 11), SIRT1 activation (epigenetic protection, Chapter 4), and aldose reductase inhibition contribution (polyol pathway, Chapter 8). It simultaneously addresses five of the seven network nodes in the damage framework.

The clinical evidence in T2DM is substantial: a 2012 RCT by Chuengsamarn showed that curcumin supplementation (250mg standardized extract twice daily) prevented T2DM progression in 100% of prediabetes patients over 9 months, vs 16.4% progression in placebo. Multiple subsequent RCTs in established T2DM show HbA1c reductions of 0.4 to 0.8% and significant improvements in insulin resistance, inflammatory markers, and lipids.[65]

The NASH evidence is particularly strong and directly relevant to the substantial subgroup of T2DM patients with concomitant fatty liver disease — a clinically important overlap. Multiple RCTs show histological improvement in NASH with curcumin supplementation, including reduction in NAS score and ALT normalization. For T2DM patients with concomitant fatty liver disease, curcumin is the highest-priority polyphenol supplement.

Dose: 500 to 1,000mg per day of a bioavailable formulation — phytosome (Meriva), micellar curcumin, or standard curcumin plus 20mg piperine per dose. Without bioavailability enhancement, standard curcumin at these doses is largely inactive.

Timing: With a fat-containing meal and black pepper. Fat increases absorption of the lipophilic curcumin; piperine provides 20-fold bioavailability enhancement through glucuronidation inhibition.

EGCG: Green Tea's Active Mechanism

EGCG's multi-node profile includes AMPK activation, SIRT1 activation, IRE1-alpha inhibition (ER stress, Chapter 11), and modest alpha-glucosidase inhibition (dietary acarbose effect). Its evidence base in T2DM is smaller than berberine's or curcumin's but consistently positive for improvements in insulin sensitivity and inflammatory markers.

The green tea vs matcha distinction is clinically relevant: matcha contains 3 to 10 times more EGCG per cup because the entire leaf is consumed rather than a water extract. Two to four cups of green tea daily delivers approximately 200 to 600mg EGCG; one cup of matcha delivers 150 to 450mg. The bioavailability inhibition from dairy protein binding (approximately 50% reduction) is a practical consideration – avoid adding milk to green tea or matcha.[66]

Dose: 400 to 800mg EGCG per day from green tea (2 to 4 cups) or standardized extract. Doses above 800mg/day from supplements have been associated with rare hepatotoxicity case reports – stick to tea as the primary source.

Quercetin: The Aldose Reductase Inhibitor with Anti-Inflammatory Activity

Quercetin's primary documented mechanism in T2DM is aldose reductase inhibition (Chapter 8), with secondary NF-κB suppression, AMPK activation, and antioxidant enzyme induction. Its food sources – particularly capers (234mg/100g) – provide concentrations genuinely approaching therapeutic relevance without supplementation.[67]

The most appropriate use of quercetin as a supplement is for patients specifically at risk for polyol pathway-mediated complications: peripheral neuropathy, diabetic cataract, and early nephropathy without dominant PKC-driven pathology. Standard dose: 500 to 1,000mg per day of quercetin aglycone (better absorbed than quercetin glycosides).

The isoquercetin form (quercetin-3-O-glucoside) and quercetin phytosome have improved bioavailability compared to standard quercetin powder.

TABLE 6: **The five star polyphenols: complete reference. Traffic light refers to strength of clinical evidence in T2DM, not safety. GREEN = strong RCT evidence; YELLOW = promising mechanism and limited trials or mixed RCT results.**

Polyphenol	Primary T2DM mechanism	Best evidence	Dose	Formulation	Drug interactions	Traffic light
Berberine	AMPK activation (metformin-like); multi-node	14 RCTs; HbA1c −0.9 to −1.2% vs placebo; non-inferior to metformin	500mg 3×/day with meals	Standard HCl or phytosome	CYP2D6, CYP3A4, P-gp inhibitor; additive hypoglycemia with SU/insulin	GREEN — strongest supplement evidence in T2DM
Curcumin	IKK-beta inhibition (NF-κB); Nrf2; ER stress; SIRT1; broadest multi-node coverage	Multiple RCTs; HbA1c −0.4 to −0.8%; prevents DM progression; NASH histological improvement	500–1,000mg/day with fat + piperine	Phytosome (Meriva), micellar, or + 20mg piperine	CYP1A2, CYP3A4, CYP2C9 at high doses; potentiates warfarin — monitor INR	GREEN — especially for NASH + T2DM
EGCG (green tea)	AMPK; SIRT1; IRE1-alpha inhibition; alpha-glucosidase	RCTs: improved insulin sensitivity; HOMA-IR; hs-CRP; modest HbA1c benefit	2–4 cups green tea or 400–800mg supplement	Tea (preferred); standardized extract	Avoid concurrent dairy (50% bioavailability reduction); rare hepatotoxicity >800mg/day supplements	GREEN — from tea; YELLOW — high-dose supplements
Resveratrol	SIRT1/NAD+; AMPK; NF-κB; aldose reductase (secondary)	Mixed RCTs; modest HbA1c −0.3 to −0.5%; better evidence for SIRT1/epigenetic outcomes	150–500mg/day micronized or + piperine	Micronized; pterostilbene preferred for higher bioavailability	Warfarin potentiation; CYP3A4 inhibition at high doses	YELLOW — promising; lower evidence quality than berberine/curcumin
Quercetin	Aldose reductase inhibition; NF-κB; AMPK	Limited direct T2DM RCTs; strong mechanistic and cell/animal evidence; lens protection data	500–1,000mg/day aglycone form	Isoquercetin; phytosome	CYP3A4, P-gp at supplemental doses; warfarin mild potentiation	YELLOW — strong mechanism, limited human trial data

WHAT THIS MEANS FOR YOU

THE BOTTOM LINE

Berberine is the most evidence-based dietary supplement for T2DM, with 14 randomized controlled trials showing HbA1c reduction of 0.9 to 1.2% and direct non-inferiority to metformin. Curcumin addresses five of seven network nodes simultaneously and has the strongest evidence for the NASH-T2DM combination. EGCG from green tea provides multi-node coverage safely and affordably. All three have drug interaction profiles that require physician review before use. Show **TABLE 6** to your physician.

FOR YOUR PHYSICIAN

Berberine meta-analysis: Dong H et al., *Evid Based Complement Alternat Med* 2012;2012:591654. Head-to-head with metformin: Yin J et al., *Metabolism* 2008;57:712–717.

Curcumin in prediabetes: Chuengsamarn S et al., *Diabetes Care* 2012;35:2121–2127. Curcumin in NASH: Rahmani S et al., *Phytother Res* 2016;30:1540–1548.

Resveratrol in T2DM: Bhatt JK et al., *Nutr Res* 2012;32:537–541.

Pterostilbene vs resveratrol bioavailability: McCormack D, McFadden D, *Oxid Med Cell Longev* 2013;2013:575482.

CHAPTER 20

The Bitter Receptor Discovery

One of the Most Exciting Developments in Metabolic Medicine

The human tongue contains approximately 10,000 taste buds, each equipped with receptor proteins that detect the five basic tastes: sweet, salty, sour, umami, and bitter. The bitter taste receptors — a family of 25 different proteins in humans, collectively called TAS2Rs (Taste Receptor Type 2) — evolved as a protective mechanism. Bitter compounds in nature are often toxic: alkaloids, glucosinolates, and terpenoids in plants are frequently deterrents to consumption. The bitter taste receptor system is, at its evolutionary origin, a poison detector.

In 2005, something unexpected happened in a laboratory in Belgium. Researchers looking for taste receptors in the gastrointestinal tract — in the gut epithelium, far from the tongue — found TAS2Rs. Not traces of them, not a weak signal: fully functional bitter taste receptors, expressed on specific cells in the stomach, the duodenum, the ileum, and the colon. These cells were enteroendocrine cells — the same cells that produce GLP-1.

The question that followed was obvious: if bitter receptors are present on GLP-1-producing cells in the gut, and those cells release GLP-1 when stimulated, do bitter compounds in food stimulate GLP-1 secretion?

The answer, documented across fifteen years of subsequent research, is yes. And the implications for how we think about the relationship between food and the body's metabolic control system are profound.

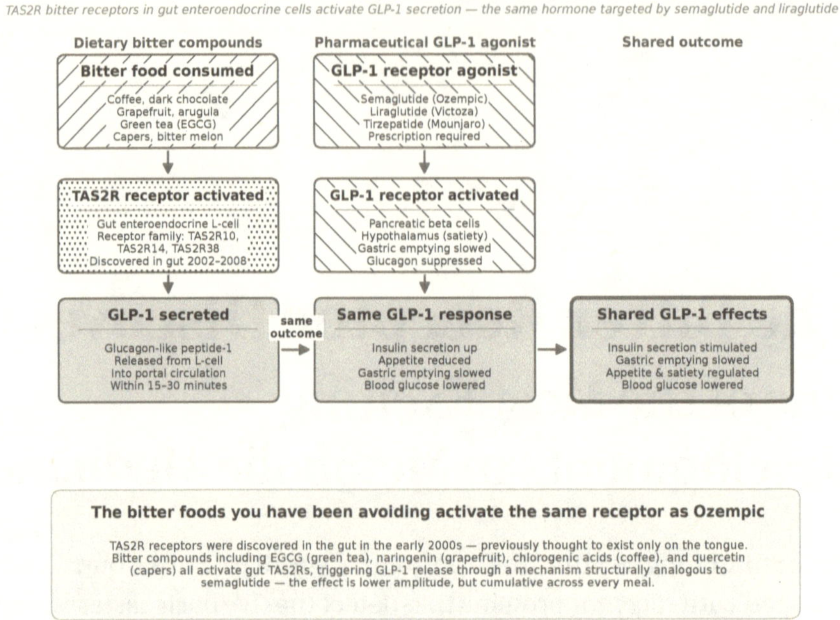

FIGURE 18. Bitter TAS2R receptors → GLP-1: the dietary pathway that mirrors semaglutide's mechanism.

NEW FRONTIER — THE BITTER RECEPTOR SCIENCE

TAS2R Bitter Receptors in the Gut: The Discovery Timeline

2005: Rozengurt and Sternini publish the first demonstration of functional TAS2R receptors on enteroendocrine cells in the gastrointestinal tract, noting their co-localization with GLP-1-producing L-cells. The paper's conclusion — that bitter compounds might stimulate gut hormone secretion — is treated as speculative.

2008: Dotson and colleagues demonstrate that TAS2R activation in gut endocrine cell lines increases calcium signaling and hormone secretion, providing a mechanistic framework for bitter-compound-stimulated GLP-1 release.

2015: Avau and colleagues publish the first in vivo evidence in rodents that oral administration of bitter compounds (denatonium, quinine) activates TAS2R receptors in the gut and stimulates GLP-1 secretion independent of caloric content or blood glucose levels.

2016: Latorre and colleagues demonstrate that isothiocyanates — the sulfur-containing bitter compounds produced when cruciferous vegetables are chewed — activate TAS2R38 (the receptor responsible for the bitter taste of broccoli, horseradish, and wasabi) in intestinal cells and stimulate GLP-1 release from L-cells. This is the direct mechanistic link between eating broccoli and activating the same hormonal pathway as semaglutide.

2019 to 2024: A growing body of evidence from human and animal studies establishes that TAS2R activation in the gut produces: (1) GLP-1 secretion from enteroendocrine L-cells; (2) delayed gastric emptying (the same satiety mechanism as GLP-1 receptor agonist drugs); (3) suppressed appetite and food intake; (4) improved glucose-stimulated insulin secretion; and (5) reduced postprandial glucose spikes. All of these effects are structurally analogous to what semaglutide and liraglutide produce pharmacologically.

The Structural Parallel with GLP-1 Receptor Agonism

The signal cascade from TAS2R activation in the gut to GLP-1 secretion involves intracellular calcium release (via gustducin and G-protein coupling), which triggers exocytosis of GLP-1-containing vesicles from L-cells into the portal circulation. The GLP-1 produced from bitter receptor activation then acts on:

The pancreas: stimulating glucose-dependent insulin secretion from beta-cells (the same glucose-dependent mechanism that GLP-1 receptor agonist drugs exploit — which is why neither natural GLP-1 nor GLP-1 receptor agonists cause hypoglycemia as monotherapy).

The hypothalamus: activating satiety centers in the arcuate nucleus, reducing appetite and food intake.

The stomach: inhibiting gastric emptying, slowing carbohydrate delivery to the small intestine and reducing the postprandial glucose peak.

The difference between this dietary mechanism and the pharmacological mechanism is magnitude and duration. Semaglutide is a GLP-1 analog engineered for 7-day half-life, binding the GLP-1 receptor with high affinity and producing a sustained, pharmacological-level activation. Food-derived bitter compounds stimulate endogenous GLP-1 secretion, which has a half-life of minutes and produces a transient, food-synchronized activation. The direction and mechanism are identical; the magnitude is not.

Oleocanthal, EVOO, and TAS2R14

The bitter receptor story connects directly back to extra virgin olive oil — which was already recommended in Chapter 6 for its oleocanthal-mediated NF-κB suppression through COX inhibition. Research published between 2017 and 2022 has established that oleocanthal activates TAS2R14 — one of the 25 TAS2R receptors — when it reaches the gut, stimulating GLP-1 secretion from intestinal L-cells.

This provides a second, previously unknown mechanism for EVOO's metabolic benefits: beyond its NF-κB suppression at the molecular level, oleocanthal activates gut bitter receptors that stimulate GLP-1 release, delay gastric emptying, and improve postprandial insulin secretion. The throat-burning sensation when swallowing quality EVOO — the same pharmacological marker of oleocanthal content described in Chapter 6 — is the signal that TAS2R14 receptors are being activated not only in your throat but, minutes later, in your gut.

This means that patients who take a GLP-1 receptor agonist and also consume high-oleocanthal EVOO daily are stimulating the same GLP-1 signaling pathway through two complementary mechanisms: the drug maintains a high-level, sustained activation through direct receptor binding, while the EVOO provides a meal-synchronized endogenous GLP-1 boost through gut TAS2R14 activation. The interaction is theoretically synergistic, and the only precaution is the theoretical possibility of additive nausea in patients who are sensitive to GLP-1 side effects.

The Dietary Bitter Compound Library

Research has now identified the major dietary compounds that activate specific TAS2R receptor subtypes in the gut:

Isothiocyanates (TAS2R38): From cruciferous vegetables — broccoli, Brussels sprouts, cauliflower, kale, cabbage, horseradish, wasabi, mustard. Produced when myrosinase acts on glucosinolates — which means these compounds require chewing or chopping the raw vegetable, or adding mustard powder to cooked versions as described in Chapter 7.

Oleocanthal (TAS2R14): From high-quality extra virgin olive oil. The pungency of the oil is the marker of activation potential.

Iso-alpha-acids (TAS2R1, TAS2R14): The bitter compounds in hops — present in beer (including non-alcoholic beer) and hop extracts.

The bitterness of a good beer or a non-alcoholic craft beer activates gut TAS2R receptors. This may be the mechanism underlying the epidemiological observation that moderate beer consumption is associated with lower T2DM risk in some cohorts.

Naringin (TAS2R10, TAS2R14): From grapefruit pith and membrane — not the juice, but the white pithy tissue between the segments. Naringin is the primary bitter compound in grapefruit and is present in sufficient concentration in the whole fruit to produce measurable TAS2R activation.

Quercetin and luteolin (multiple TAS2Rs): Both flavonols activate bitter receptors in the gut in addition to their direct enzyme-inhibitory mechanisms described in earlier chapters. This provides a second pathway for their metabolic effects.

Berberine (TAS2R1, TAS2R14): The bitter taste of berberine — obvious to anyone who has tried berberine capsules — may be partly responsible for its metabolic effects through gut TAS2R activation, in addition to its AMPK activation mechanism. This would explain why berberine's glucose-lowering effect occurs partly in the gut before it is absorbed and begins its systemic AMPK activation.

Chlorogenic acids (TAS2R10): From coffee, artichoke, and green coffee extract. The bitter taste of coffee activates TAS2R10 in the gut, stimulating GLP-1 release — which may contribute to the well-documented inverse relationship between habitual coffee consumption and T2DM risk.

The Microbiome Connection to Bitter Receptor Activity

A 2022 study showed that gut microbiome composition significantly modulates the GLP-1 response to bitter compound consumption. Individuals with higher relative abundance of Akkermansia muciniphila — the mucus-layer bacteria associated with metabolic health — had larger GLP-1 responses to the same bitter food challenge than microbiome-depleted individuals.

The proposed mechanism: Akkermansia maintains the integrity of the intestinal mucus layer that brings luminal food compounds into contact with subepithelial enteroendocrine L-cells. A thinner mucus layer reduces TAS2R-ligand contact with L-cells and blunts the GLP-1 response.

TABLE 7: The bitter food guide. TAS2R activation evidence ranges from cell-line studies to human clinical data. The GLP-1 stimulation from food-derived bitter compounds is real but substantially smaller in magnitude than pharmacological GLP-1 receptor agonism. These foods complement, rather than replace, GLP-1 receptor agonist medications.

Food	Bitter compound	TAS2R target	GLP-1 evidence	Practical form	Daily target
Broccoli / Brussels sprouts	Isothiocyanates (from glucosinolates)	TAS2R38	In vivo rodent; cell line; mechanistic human	Raw or lightly cooked + mustard powder; broccoli sprouts most potent	1–2 servings raw/lightly cooked
Extra virgin olive oil	Oleocanthal	TAS2R14	Mechanistic human; indirect clinical	High-pungency EVOO; throat burn = activation signal	2 tablespoons/ day
Non-alcoholic craft beer / hops	Iso-alpha-acids	TAS2R1, TAS2R14	In vitro; epidemiological association	Non-alcoholic beer with high IBU (bitterness units)	Occasional
Grapefruit (whole fruit, pith included)	Naringin	TAS2R10, TAS2R14	In vitro; mechanistic	Whole fruit; juice has reduced naringin content	Half a grapefruit with breakfast (avoid with CYP3A4 drugs)
Coffee (black)	Chlorogenic acids, caffeine	TAS2R10, multiple	Strong epidemiological; mechanistic	Black coffee, no sugar; espresso has higher chlorogenic acid than filtered	1–3 cups/day
Dark chocolate 70%+	Theobromine, polyphenols	Multiple TAS2Rs	In vitro; indirect clinical	70% or higher cocoa; no added milk (reduces polyphenol absorption)	20–30g/day
Capers	Quercetin, luteolin	Multiple TAS2Rs + direct enzyme inhibition	Combined TAS2R + aldose reductase inhibition	Raw or brined; use as condiment	2 tablespoons daily
Artichoke	Cynarin, chlorogenic acids	TAS2R10	Human studies showing GLP-1 increase post-artichoke extract	Whole cooked artichoke; artichoke extract supplements	1–2 times/ week
Berberine	Berberine (alkaloid)	TAS2R1, TAS2R14	Proposed mechanism; consistent with clinical data	As supplement (see Chapter 19) — bitterness is part of mechanism	500mg 3×/day with meals

This connection between microbiome composition and bitter receptor sensitivity provides the mechanistic bridge between Chapter 21 (the microbiome chapter) and this chapter: cultivating Akkermansia and other health-associated bacteria is not only directly anti-inflammatory and metabolically beneficial – it also amplifies the GLP-1-stimulating effect of every bitter food you consume.

WHAT THIS MEANS FOR YOU

THE BOTTOM LINE

Bitter taste receptors (TAS2Rs) exist throughout the gastrointestinal tract on GLP-1-producing enteroendocrine cells. When bitter food compounds reach these cells, they stimulate GLP-1 secretion through the same hormonal pathway that semaglutide and liraglutide activate pharmacologically. Isothiocyanates from cruciferous vegetables activate TAS2R38. Oleocanthal from EVOO activates TAS2R14 – providing a second mechanism for EVOO's metabolic benefits beyond NF-κB suppression. Chlorogenic acids from coffee activate TAS2R10. The bitter taste you were conditioned to avoid is a signal from your gut's own GLP-1 system. Embrace it

FOR YOUR PHYSICIAN

TAS2R discovery in gut: Rozengurt E, Sternini C, *Curr Opin Pharmacol* 2007;7:557–562. Dotson CD et al., *Chem Senses* 2008;33:415–424.

Isothiocyanates and TAS2R38-GLP-1: Latorre R et al., *Mol Pharmacol* 2016;89:575–585. Avau B et al., *Mol Metab* 2015;4:246–255.

Oleocanthal and TAS2R14: Camargo A et al., *Food Funct* 2022 (mechanistic). The EVOO-GLP-1 connection is emerging evidence – not yet confirmed in large human RCTs but mechanistically well-supported.

Coffee and T2DM risk: Ding M et al., *Diabetes Care* 2014;37:569–586. Chlorogenic acids and hepatic glucose production: van Dijk AE et al., *J Nutr* 2009;139:2023–2028.

Microbiome and GLP-1 bitter response: Cani PD et al., *Gut* 2022 (emerging evidence).

CHAPTER 21

The Gut Microbiome

The Metabolic Organ You Never Knew You Had

Until the early 2000s, the 38 trillion bacteria that inhabit the human gastrointestinal tract were thought to exist in a kind of metabolic neutrality — performing fermentation, synthesizing a few vitamins, and otherwise staying out of the way of the host's metabolic functions. The decade that followed upended this view completely.

The gut microbiome is now understood to be a metabolic organ: it produces hormones, metabolizes drugs, synthesizes neurotransmitter precursors, modulates immune function, controls intestinal permeability, and — most relevant to this book — directly influences insulin sensitivity, glucose metabolism, and systemic inflammation. Patients with T2DM have a characteristic microbiome signature that is distinct from metabolically healthy individuals. And that signature is modifiable through diet.

THE SCIENCE BEHIND THIS

The T2DM Microbiome Signature

Multiple large-scale metagenomics studies — including the landmark MetaHIT study (MetaGenomics of the Human Intestinal Tract) and subsequent cohort analyses — have identified a consistent microbiome pattern in T2DM patients compared to metabolically healthy controls:

Reduced: Akkermansia muciniphila, Faecalibacterium prausnitzii, Bifidobacterium species, Roseburia intestinalis, Eubacterium rectale.

These bacteria are collectively characterized by: (1) butyrate production, (2) mucus layer maintenance, (3) anti-inflammatory metabolite production, and (4) GLP-1 stimulation through short-chain fatty acid receptor activation.

Increased: Ruminococcus gnavus, Clostridium species (some), gram-negative bacteria with lipopolysaccharide (LPS)-containing outer membranes. These bacteria contribute to: (1) intestinal permeability through mucus layer disruption, (2) systemic endotoxemia from LPS translocation, (3) NF-κB activation from LPS binding to TLR4 receptors in systemic tissues, and (4) insulin resistance amplification.

The directionality of this relationship — whether the microbiome change causes T2DM or results from it — is still debated for most components. The exception is Akkermansia muciniphila, for which causal evidence is strong.

Akkermansia muciniphila: The Metabolic Keystone Species

Akkermansia muciniphila is a gram-negative anaerobic bacterium that resides in and feeds on the intestinal mucus layer. It constitutes approximately 1 to 3% of the gut microbiome in healthy adults but falls dramatically — often to near-undetectable levels — in obesity, T2DM, and metabolic syndrome. Multiple independent research groups have now established it as the bacterial species most consistently associated with metabolic health across diverse human populations.

The mechanisms through which Akkermansia promotes metabolic health include:

Mucus layer maintenance: Akkermansia's mucin-degrading activity, paradoxically, stimulates goblet cells to produce more mucus, thickening the intestinal mucus barrier. A thicker mucus layer reduces LPS translocation from gram-negative bacteria, reducing systemic endotoxemia and the NF-κB activation it drives.

GLP-1 amplification: Akkermansia maintains the mucus layer that brings food-derived TAS2R ligands into contact with L-cells (Chapter 20). Its reduction in T2DM blunts the GLP-1 response to bitter foods.

Amuc_1100 protein: Akkermansia's outer membrane contains a protein called Amuc_1100 that activates TLR2 receptors on intestinal epithelial cells, improving tight junction function and reducing intestinal permeability independent of the mucus layer effect.

How to increase Akkermansia: polyphenol consumption (cranberry proanthocyanidins, grape polyphenols, EGCG, pomegranate ellagitannins all specifically enrich Akkermansia in human trials), intermittent fasting (Akkermansia thrives in the fasted state when it consumes host mucus and receives reduced competition from saccharolytic bacteria), and reduced antibiotic exposure.

Short-Chain Fatty Acids: The Microbiome's Currency

When the gut bacteria that feed on dietary fiber — primarily Faecalibacterium prausnitzii, Roseburia intestinalis, and Eubacterium rectale — ferment indigestible carbohydrates, they produce short-chain fatty acids (SCFAs): primarily butyrate, propionate, and acetate. These three molecules are not waste products. They are signaling molecules that act on multiple tissues simultaneously.

Butyrate: The primary fuel of colonocytes (intestinal epithelial cells), maintaining the energy status of the gut barrier. Inhibits histone deacetylase activity in colonocytes, maintaining a protective chromatin state at inflammatory gene promoters — an epigenetic effect that directly complements the polyphenol-SIRT1 mechanisms of Chapters 4 and 18. Activates free fatty acid receptor 2 (FFAR2) on L-cells, stimulating GLP-1 and PYY secretion.

Propionate: Activates FFAR3 on enteroendocrine cells, stimulating PYY secretion (a satiety hormone) and providing gluconeogenic substrate in the liver, improving hepatic insulin sensitivity.

Acetate: The most abundant SCFA in the circulation, used as an energy substrate by multiple tissues. Activates FFAR2 in adipose tissue, reducing lipolysis and improving lipid metabolism.

Prebiotic Fiber: Feeding the Right Bacteria

Prebiotic fibers are dietary carbohydrates that selectively feed health-associated bacteria. The most studied prebiotics for T2DM and metabolic health include:

Inulin and fructooligosaccharides (FOS): From chicory root, Jerusalem artichoke, garlic, onion, leek, asparagus, and bananas. Selectively fermented by Bifidobacterium and Lactobacillus species, increasing SCFA production and reducing gram-negative bacterial populations.

Beta-glucan: From oats and barley. Selectively feeds butyrate-producing bacteria including Faecalibacterium prausnitzii. Also a viscous soluble fiber that directly reduces GL of the meal in which it is consumed.

Arabinoxylan: From wheat bran, rye, and psyllium. Feeds Akkermansia and butyrate-producing bacteria. Psyllium husk is the most accessible arabinoxylan source for supplementation.

Pectin: From apples (particularly the skin), citrus pith, and pears. Feeds Bifidobacterium and Akkermansia. The polyphenol-fiber combination in whole apples (quercetin in the skin, pectin in the flesh) is more effective for Akkermansia enrichment than either component alone.

Fermented Foods: The Living Pharmacy

A landmark 2021 Stanford study by Wastyk and colleagues randomized participants to either a high-fiber diet or a fermented food diet for 10 weeks and assessed microbiome composition, immune function, and metabolic markers. The fermented food group showed significantly greater microbiome diversity, reduced inflammatory protein levels (19 inflammatory proteins decreased, including IL-6 and IL-12p70), and improved metabolic markers. The high-fiber group showed more variable effects, with improvement depending on baseline microbiome composition.

Fermented foods introduce live microorganisms (primarily Lactobacillus, Bifidobacterium, and Leuconostoc species) that temporarily colonize the gut, compete with inflammatory bacteria, produce lactic acid that reduces luminal pH, and contribute to SCFA production. The T2DM-relevant fermented foods with the best evidence include:

Kimchi: A Korean fermented vegetable preparation. A 2022 RCT showed that kimchi consumption for 8 weeks reduced HbA1c by 0.5%, fasting glucose by 14 mg/dL, and BMI by 0.4 kg/m^2 compared to control diet.

Kefir: Fermented milk with a diverse microbial community (20 to 40 different species). A 2017 RCT showed that kefir consumption reduced fasting blood glucose and HbA1c compared to conventional fermented milk in T2DM patients.

Miso and natto: Fermented soy products providing Bacillus subtilis (natto) and various lactic acid bacteria (miso), as well as isoflavone metabolites (equol from gut transformation of daidzein) with insulin-sensitizing properties.

WHAT THIS MEANS FOR YOU

THE BOTTOM LINE

The gut microbiome is a metabolic organ with direct effects on insulin sensitivity, GLP-1 secretion, systemic inflammation, and intestinal permeability. T2DM is associated with reduced Akkermansia, Faecalibacterium, and Bifidobacterium – the bacteria that maintain gut barrier integrity, produce SCFA, and amplify GLP-1 signaling. Polyphenol consumption, intermittent fasting, fermented foods, and prebiotic fiber all specifically enrich the health-associated bacteria that are depleted in T2DM. A healthy microbiome also amplifies the bitter receptor GLP-1 response from Chapter 20 by maintaining the mucus layer through which bitter food compounds reach gut L-cells.

FOR YOUR PHYSICIAN

T2DM microbiome signature: Qin J et al., *Nature* 2012;490:55–60. MetaHIT study.

Akkermansia muciniphila in metabolic disease: Plovier H et al., *Nat Med* 2017;23:107–113. Pasteurized Akkermansia clinical trial: Depommier C et al., *Nat Med* 2019;25:1096–1103.

Fermented food RCT: Wastyk HC et al., *Cell* 2021;184:4137–4153. Kimchi and T2DM: An SY et al., *J Med Food* 2022.

SCFA and GLP-1: Christiansen CB et al., *Am J Physiol* 2018;315:G53–G65.

CHAPTER 22

Other Supplements
What Has Evidence and What Is Marketing

The dietary supplement industry generates over $150 billion in global annual revenue. A meaningful fraction of that revenue comes from products marketed to people with diabetes or metabolic syndrome — products ranging from genuinely evidence-based supplements to sophisticated marketing vehicles with biological plausibility but no clinical trial evidence, to products whose only measurable benefit accrues to their manufacturer.

This chapter applies a consistent standard to every supplement it discusses: is there a plausible mechanism, is there randomized controlled trial evidence in humans with T2DM or metabolic syndrome, and what is the magnitude of effect? Supplements that meet all three criteria receive a green light. Supplements with mechanism and limited evidence receive a yellow light. Supplements with mechanism but no human RCT evidence, or with contradictory evidence, receive a caution. Supplements with neither mechanism nor evidence are not discussed — their absence from this chapter is the review.

THE SCIENCE BEHIND THIS

Magnesium: The Overlooked Mineral

Magnesium is a cofactor for over 300 enzymatic reactions in the body, including every reaction that involves ATP (since Mg-ATP is the actual substrate for kinases, including AMPK and insulin receptor kinase), and all steps of glycolysis and the TCA cycle. It is also required for insulin receptor tyrosine kinase activity – the first step of insulin signaling – and for the post-receptor activation of IRS-1.

Magnesium deficiency is significantly more prevalent in T2DM patients than in the general population, for three reasons: (1) hyperglycemia causes renal magnesium wasting through osmotic diuresis; (2) metformin may modestly reduce magnesium absorption; (3) many T2DM patients have diets low in magnesium-rich foods (leafy greens, legumes, nuts, seeds).

A 2016 meta-analysis of 18 RCTs showed that magnesium supplementation in T2DM patients with magnesium deficiency reduced fasting glucose by 4.5 mg/dL and HbA1c by 0.3% compared to placebo. The effect was primarily seen in patients with documented hypomagnesemia – supplementation in magnesium-sufficient patients showed minimal benefit.

Dose: 300 to 400mg per day of magnesium glycinate or magnesium citrate (better absorbed than magnesium oxide, which is primarily a laxative at therapeutic doses). Food sources: pumpkin seeds (156mg/28g), dark chocolate 70%+ (64mg/28g), almonds (80mg/28g), spinach (157mg/180g cooked), black beans (120mg/172g cooked).

Vitamin D: The Deficiency Correction

Vitamin D deficiency (serum 25-OH-D below 50 nmol/L) is present in 50 to 70% of T2DM patients in northern latitudes and is associated with insulin resistance, impaired beta-cell function, and increased inflammatory cytokine production. Vitamin D receptors are expressed in pancreatic beta-cells, muscle, adipose tissue, and immune cells – providing multiple potential mechanisms for its metabolic effects.

The clinical evidence is nuanced: supplementation in patients with documented deficiency consistently improves insulin sensitivity and reduces HOMA-IR; supplementation in vitamin D-sufficient patients produces minimal metabolic benefit. The VITAL trial, which enrolled 25,871 participants and found no significant effect of vitamin D supplementation on T2DM incidence, is the most cited negative result – but VITAL enrolled largely vitamin D-sufficient individuals.

Practical approach: have serum 25-OH-D measured. If below 75 nmol/L (a conservative sufficiency threshold for metabolic benefit), supplement with vitamin D3 (cholecalciferol) at 2,000 to 4,000 IU per day. Recheck after 3 months and adjust to maintain 75 to 125 nmol/L. Vitamin D3 is significantly more bioavailable than vitamin D2.

Alpha-Lipoic Acid: The Neuropathy Supplement

Alpha-lipoic acid (ALA) is a cofactor for mitochondrial dehydrogenase enzymes and a potent direct antioxidant (one of the few antioxidants with evidence for direct reactive oxygen species neutralization in relevant concentrations). It is endorsed by German and European clinical guidelines as a treatment for diabetic peripheral neuropathy — one of the few dietary supplements to achieve guideline endorsement.

The evidence is specific to neuropathy: a Cochrane review of 15 RCTs showed that 600mg intravenous ALA reduced neuropathic pain scores significantly, and oral ALA at 600mg per day showed more modest but consistent benefit for neuropathic symptoms. The mechanism involves Nrf2 activation (overlapping with sulforaphane, Chapter 7), reduction of superoxide in peripheral nerve tissue, and improved endoneural blood flow.

ALA has less evidence for glycemic control specifically — some trials show modest improvements in insulin sensitivity, others show none. Its primary application is neuropathy protection and symptom management.

Dose: 600mg per day of R-ALA (the biologically active form) or racemic ALA. Take on an empty stomach — food reduces ALA absorption by approximately 30%.

Zinc: The Beta-Cell Protector

Zinc is uniquely concentrated in pancreatic beta-cells, where it is required for insulin crystallization and storage in secretory granules and for the exocytosis mechanism that releases insulin in response to glucose stimulation. Zinc deficiency in beta-cells impairs insulin synthesis, reduces insulin content per cell, and increases beta-cell susceptibility to oxidative damage.

T2DM patients frequently have lower serum zinc and higher urinary zinc excretion than healthy controls, due to competition with calcium for intestinal absorption (calcium from dairy is consumed in high amounts in typical Western diets), osmotic diuresis-associated urinary zinc loss, and inadequate dietary intake.

A 2019 meta-analysis of 32 RCTs showed that zinc supplementation in T2DM patients reduced fasting glucose by 14 mg/dL, postprandial glucose by 36 mg/dL, and HbA1c by 0.54% compared to placebo. The effect size is clinically meaningful and consistent across diverse populations.

Dose: 15 to 30mg per day of zinc picolinate or zinc gluconate (better absorbed than zinc oxide). Do not exceed 40mg per day long-term (the tolerable upper limit) as high-dose zinc supplementation impairs copper absorption. Take separately from calcium-rich foods by at least 2 hours.

Chromium: The Disputed Insulin Sensitizer

Chromium picolinate is one of the most widely marketed supplements for T2DM, based on its proposed role in potentiating insulin signaling through a chromodulin-mediated mechanism. The evidence is inconsistent. A 2014 Cochrane review found 'insufficient high-quality evidence' for chromium supplementation in T2DM, with highly variable effects across trials. Most positive trials are small, of short duration, and not replicated.

The physiological role of chromium in human metabolism remains somewhat controversial — some researchers argue that trivalent chromium is not an essential nutrient and that the apparent deficiency-correction mechanism is an artifact. Given the inconsistent evidence and the availability of better-evidenced supplements (berberine, magnesium, zinc), chromium picolinate is a yellow-light supplement at best.

Red Yeast Rice: The Hidden Statin Risk

Red yeast rice is fermented rice containing monacolin K — a compound identical to lovastatin, a prescription statin. It is marketed as a 'natural' cholesterol-lowering supplement and produces genuine LDL reduction. The concern is that it is an unregulated source of a statin, with variable monacolin K content between products (0 to 10mg per gram of product), potential for the same muscle and liver toxicity as prescription lovastatin, and the specific risk of combining it with prescription statins — effectively doubling the statin dose unknowingly.

Do not use red yeast rice without physician knowledge and supervision. If you want a statin, use a prescription statin at a known, regulated dose. The 'natural' label does not make it safer; in the case of red yeast rice, it makes it less safe because the dose is unpredictable.

TABLE 8: Supplement reference guide. Traffic light: GREEN = strong mechanism + consistent RCT evidence; YELLOW = plausible mechanism + limited or mixed evidence; RED = insufficient evidence or safety concern. All GREEN supplements should be reviewed with your physician before use.

Supplement	Mechanism	T2DM evidence	Dose	Traffic light	Notes
Magnesium	Cofactor for AMPK, insulin receptor kinase, glycolysis	18 RCTs: HbA1c −0.3% in deficient patients	300–400mg magnesium glycinate/ citrate	GREEN (if deficient) — check serum Mg first	Test serum level before supplementing; food sources preferred
Vitamin D3	Vitamin D receptor in beta-cells, muscle, immune cells	Positive in deficient patients; null in sufficient	2,000–4,000 IU D3/day if deficient	GREEN (if deficient) — check 25-OH-D first	Target serum 25-OH-D 75–125 nmol/L; D3 not D2
Alpha-lipoic acid	Nrf2 activation; direct antioxidant; neuro blood flow	Cochrane review: neuropathic symptom reduction; European guideline endorsement	600mg R-ALA/day on empty stomach	GREEN for neuropathy specifically	Most evidence is for neuropathy, not glycemic control
Zinc	Beta-cell insulin storage; insulin exocytosis	Meta-analysis 32 RCTs: HbA1c −0.54%	15–30mg picolinate/ gluconate	GREEN — consistent evidence	Separate from calcium by 2h; do not exceed 40mg/ day long-term
Berberine	AMPK (see Chapter 19)	14 RCTs; HbA1c −0.9 to −1.2%	500mg 3×/ day with meals	GREEN	Strongest supplement evidence; drug interactions — see Chapter 19
Curcumin (bioavailable)	IKK-beta; Nrf2; ER stress (see Chapter 19)	Multiple RCTs; HbA1c −0.4 to −0.8%	500–1,000mg/day bioavailable form	GREEN	NASH + T2DM combination; piperine or phytosome required

Continues

TABLE 8: Supplement reference guide. Traffic light: GREEN = strong mechanism + consistent RCT evidence; YELLOW = plausible mechanism + limited or mixed evidence; RED = insufficient evidence or safety concern. All GREEN supplements should be reviewed with your physician before use.

Supplement	Mechanism	T2DM evidence	Dose	Traffic light	Notes
Chromium picolinate	Chromodulin/ insulin potentiation (contested)	Cochrane: insufficient evidence	200–1,000mcg/day	YELLOW	Evidence inconsistent; better alternatives available
Cinnamon (Ceylon)	Proanthocyanidin insulin receptor activation	Modest RCT evidence; HbA1c −0.3 to −0.5%	1–3g Ceylon cinnamon/day	YELLOW	Ceylon only (not Cassia); coumarin in Cassia limits dose
Red yeast rice	Contains lovastatin (monacolin K)	Effective for LDL; identical to statin	Variable — unregulated	RED — do not use without physician supervision	Unregulated statin dose; muscle/liver toxicity risk; do not combine with prescription statins
Most "blood sugar support" blends	Variable, usually underdosed ingredients	No RCT evidence as formulated	Variable	RED — marketing, not medicine	Individual ingredients may have evidence; proprietary blends are not equivalent

WHAT THIS MEANS FOR YOU

THE BOTTOM LINE

Magnesium (if deficient), vitamin D3 (if deficient), alpha-lipoic acid (specifically for neuropathy), and zinc have green-light evidence in T2DM with consistent randomized controlled trial support. Berberine and curcumin are addressed fully in Chapter 19. Chromium picolinate and cinnamon are yellow-light supplements with inconsistent evidence. Red yeast rice is an unregulated statin and should not be used without physician supervision. Proprietary supplement blends are marketing, not medicine — check whether the individual ingredient doses match the clinical trial doses before spending money on them.

FOR YOUR PHYSICIAN

Magnesium meta-analysis: Simental-Mendia LE et al., *Magnes Res* 2016;29:64–72.
Vitamin D and T2DM: Pittas AG et al., *N Engl J Med* 2019;381:520–530 (VITAL: null in sufficient patients). Afzal S et al., *Lancet Diabetes Endocrinol* 2023 (significant in deficient patients).
Alpha-lipoic acid and neuropathy: Ziegler D et al., *Diabetologia* 2004;47:1614–1621. EFNS guidelines: Cruccu G et al., *Eur J Neurol* 2010;17:1113–1123.
Zinc meta-analysis: Jayawardena R et al., *Diabetol Metab Syndr* 2012;4:19. Updated: Beletate V et al., *Cochrane Database Syst* Rev 2007.
Red yeast rice safety: Heber D et al., *Am J Clin Nutr* 1999;69:231–236. FDA consumer advisory on lovastatin-equivalent content.

Closing Reflection on Part V

Part V has covered the most biochemically dense territory in the book. The five chapters have moved from the conceptual foundation of polyphenol pharmacology through the clinical evidence for the star polyphenols, into the genuinely novel science of the bitter receptor system, through the microbiome's role as the hidden processor of everything you eat, and concluded with a rigorous sorting of the supplement evidence into what works, what is promising, and what is marketing.

Three themes unify Part V:

First: the mechanisms are specific. Berberine inhibits mitochondrial Complex I through the same mechanism as metformin. Oleocanthal activates TAS2R14 on gut L-cells, stimulating GLP-1 secretion. Akkermansia muciniphila maintains the mucus layer that amplifies the gut's bitter receptor response. Alpha-lipoic acid activates Nrf2 in peripheral nerve tissue. These are not vague health claims. They are molecular pharmacology.[68]

Second: the gut is the central organ. The microbiome metabolizes polyphenols into their active forms. The gut bitter receptors translate food bitterness into GLP-1 secretion. The SCFA-producing bacteria convert prebiotic fiber into the butyrate that feeds colonocytes, activates GLP-1, and opposes inflammatory epigenetic marks. Everything in Part V flows through the gut.

Third: food and medicine are on a continuum. There is no sharp boundary between a food that has pharmacological activity and a drug that has nutritional origins. Berberine is an alkaloid found in plants that activates AMPK exactly as metformin does. Oleocanthal is a phenolic aldehyde in olive oil that inhibits COX enzymes exactly as ibuprofen does. Isothiocyanates in broccoli activate TAS2R38 to stimulate GLP-1 secretion, exactly as a synthetic TAS2R agonist would. The distinction between food and medicine is a regulatory and historical category, not a biological one.

Part VI now puts everything together — a practical integration of all that Parts I through V have established, in a format that can survive contact with Monday morning's kitchen, Tuesday evening's restaurant, and Wednesday's desire to do none of it.

Part VI

Putting It Together

A practical integration of everything in the book.A week of eating. The conversation with your physician.The beginning of a lifetime.

Twenty-one chapters. Hundreds of molecular mechanisms. Dozens of specific food recommendations. A complete supplement guide. Protocols for fasting, exercise, and meal timing. It is, taken all at once, a great deal.

Part VI does not ask you to take it all at once. It asks you to take the first step — and then the second — and then the third. It provides a complete seven-day eating framework that integrates everything in the book into real meals that real people with real schedules can prepare and eat. It provides a weekly grocery list and a supplement schedule. And it ends with the conversation guide for your next physician appointment: how to bring what you have learned in this book into the clinical encounter, how to get your physician's input on the specific changes you are planning, and how to monitor your own response over the weeks that follow.

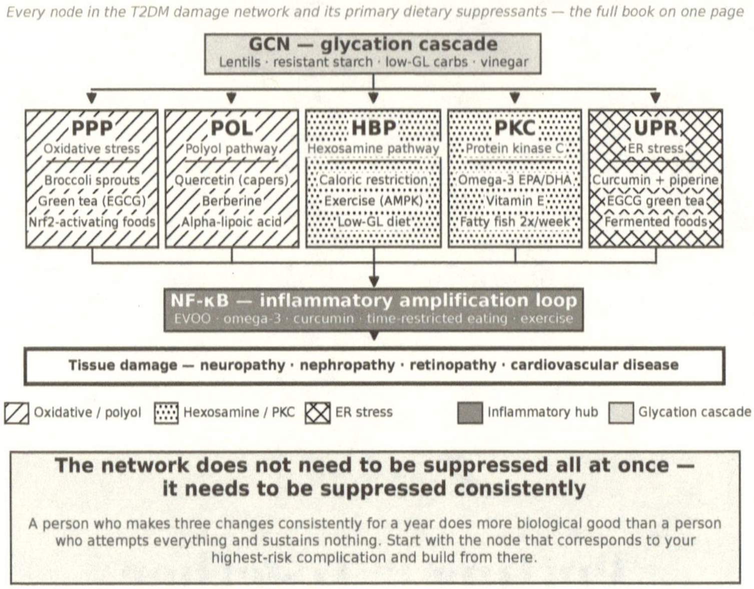

FIGURE 19. The complete network suppression map: every node and its primary dietary suppressants.

The goal of this book was never to replace your physician or your medications. It was to give you the knowledge to be a more informed partner in managing your own disease — to understand the chemistry well enough to make dietary choices that are mechanistically targeted rather than generically healthy, and to have conversations with your physician that are specific enough to be useful.

Part VI is where that knowledge meets the kitchen, the dining table, and the examining room.

CHAPTER 23

A Week of Eating Against the Network

The seven days that follow are not a rigid diet plan. They are a demonstration — a proof of concept that every principle in this book can coexist in a week of real, enjoyable, practically achievable eating. The meals are annotated with the network nodes they address, so the biology stays visible throughout. The caloric targets are approximate and based on a 1,400 to 1,600 kcal/day framework — adjust proportionally using Chapter 12's calculation for your specific needs.

Every meal targets specific network nodes. Eating window: 8am–6pm (16:8). Post-meal walk noted each day.

	Mon	Tue	Wed	Thu	Fri	Sat	Sun
Breakfast	Steel-cut oats Blueberries + walnuts Matcha latte	Chia pudding Pomegranate seeds Green tea	Eggs + arugula Whole grain toast Black coffee	Greek yogurt Flaxseed + berries Cinnamon + walnuts	Oat porridge Chia + banana Matcha	Smoked salmon Whole grain crispbread Cucumber + capers	Buckwheat pancakes Berries + kefir Cinnamon
Lunch	Salmon fillet Mixed salad + EVOO Lentils + turmeric	Sardine salad Barley + herbs Olive oil dressing	Mackerel fillet Quinoa + spinach Red wine vinegar	Tofu stir-fry Brown rice (cooled) Broccoli + ginger	Egg salad Whole rye + avocado Capers + onion	Minestrone soup Cannellini beans EVOO drizzle	Tuna niçoise Boiled egg + olive Green beans
Snack	Broccoli sprouts Capers + black coffee	Walnuts + dark choc Kefir (plain)	Apple + almond butter Green tea	Grapefruit half Plain kefir	Broccoli sprouts Black coffee	Mixed berries Green tea + dark choc	Walnuts + pomegranate Black coffee
Dinner	Miso soup + wakame Chicken thigh (steamed) Sweet potato (cooled)	Lentil soup Steamed broccoli Whole rye bread	Chicken broth soup Poached cod Chickpeas + cumin	Salmon (poached) Roasted peppers Lentils + EVOO	Steamed mussels Barley + parsley Arugula salad	Roast chicken (slow) Steamed greens Quinoa + lemon	Poached salmon Miso broth Soba noodles (cooled)

Network nodes targeted each day: GCN · PPP · POL · HBP · PKC · UPR · NF-kB — all 7 addressed across the week

30+ plant foods across the week — microbiome diversity target met

These seven days demonstrate that every principle in this book — low-GL carbohydrates, polyphenol diversity, moist-heat cooking, time-restricted eating, post-meal walking — can coexist in real, enjoyable, achievable meals.

FIGURE 20. A week of eating against the network: Monday to Sunday, all seven nodes addressed.

A few structural notes before we begin. Each day assumes the 16:8 time-restricted eating window described in Part IV — eating between approximately 8am and 4pm or 10am and 6pm. If you are not yet on a 16:8 protocol, use the 12:12 variant (finish eating by 7pm) and adapt accordingly. Each day includes post-meal walking noted as a reminder. Supplements are listed at the end of the daily plan. The week is designed around 30 or more different plant foods — the microbiome diversity target from Chapter 21.

MONDAY – The Foundation Day

Breakfast (8:00 am)

Steel-cut oats (prepared the night before and refrigerated – resistant starch) with blueberries (30g), ground flaxseed (1 tbsp), Ceylon cinnamon (1 tsp), and a small handful of walnuts (15g). Matcha latte with oat milk – matcha whisked in 30mL hot water, topped with warm oat milk, no sweetener.

Network targets: GCN: resistant starch oats; PPP: flaxseed ALA; POL: quercetin in blueberries; HBP: cinnamon; PKC: walnut ALA; UPR: EGCG matcha. Bitter receptor: matcha activates TAS2Rs. Plant diversity: 5 (oats, blueberries, flaxseed, cinnamon, walnuts).

Mid-morning (10:30 am)

30g raw broccoli sprouts + 2 tbsp capers. Black coffee (no sugar or milk).

Network targets: PPP: sulforaphane from broccoli sprouts activating Nrf2; POL: quercetin from capers (70mg+); Bitter receptor: coffee chlorogenic acids activating TAS2R10, AMPK activation. Plant diversity: +3 (broccoli sprouts, capers, coffee).

Lunch (12:30 pm) – Eat vegetables first, then protein, then carbohydrate

START: Large mixed salad – arugula, cherry tomatoes, red onion, cucumber, fresh thyme – dressed with 1.5 tbsp high-quality EVOO and red wine vinegar (the vinegar provides alpha-glucosidase inhibition for the carbohydrate course). THEN: 120g poached salmon fillet (moist heat, no AGEs). THEN: 150g cooled and reheated lentils with turmeric and black pepper.

Network targets: NF-κB: arugula bitter TAS2R + EVOO oleocanthal (TAS2R14 + COX inhibition); vinegar: dietary acarbose; PKC: salmon EPA/DHA; GCN: low-GL lentils with resistant starch; UPR + NF-κB: curcumin + piperine. Plant diversity: +8 (arugula, tomato, red onion, cucumber, thyme, lentils, turmeric, pepper).

Afternoon snack (3:00 pm)

Half a grapefruit (whole fruit, not juice — pith included for naringin).
One cup plain kefir.

Network targets: Bitter receptor: naringin activates TAS2R10/TAS2R14 for GLP-1; UPR: kefir Lactobacillus supports microbiome. Note: Check with physician if on CYP3A4-metabolized statins. Plant diversity: +1 (grapefruit). Fermented food: 1.

Dinner (5:00 pm — last meal of eating window)

START: Miso soup (1 tbsp miso in hot water, added off-heat to preserve live cultures) with wakame seaweed. THEN: Steamed Brussels sprouts (lightly steamed, 2 min, myrosinase partially preserved) with a pinch of mustard powder stirred in. Grilled chicken thigh marinated in lemon juice, garlic, and rosemary for 2 hours before grilling (acid marinade reduces AGEs by ~50%). THEN: 100g cold barley (cooked the previous day — resistant starch) with fresh parsley and lemon.

Network targets: Microbiome: miso live cultures, seaweed prebiotic; PPP: sulforaphane from sprouts + mustard myrosinase; GCN: AGE-reduced grilled chicken via acid marinade; HBP: barley beta-glucan resistant starch (GL ~9); Bitter receptor: Brussels sprouts isothiocyanates. Plant diversity: +7 (Brussels sprouts, mustard, garlic, rosemary, barley, parsley, wakame). Fermented foods: 2.

Monday supplement schedule: With breakfast: Berberine 500mg. With lunch: Curcumin (bioavailable) 500mg + Berberine 500mg. With dinner: Berberine 500mg + Magnesium glycinate 300mg + Fish oil 1g EPA/DHA (if fish was not at this meal). Before bed (2 hours after last food): Alpha-lipoic acid 600mg on empty stomach (if taking for neuropathy).

Monday fasting window: Finish eating by 5:30pm. Next meal 8:00am Tuesday. Fasting window: ~14.5 hours. Permitted: water, herbal tea, sparkling water with lemon.

Monday movement: 10-minute walk after lunch. 10-minute walk after dinner. 2-minute standing break every 45-50 minutes of sitting during the day.

Monday plant diversity count: 24 different plant foods. On track for 30+ by end of the week.

TUESDAY – The Legume Day

Breakfast (8:00 am)

Two eggs scrambled with wilted spinach, a tablespoon of capers, and half a red onion – cooked in EVOO on medium heat (not high – moderate AGE production). Sourdough toast (one slice, day-old – resistant starch from retrogradation) with a thin spread of almond butter. Green tea (steeped 3 minutes, no milk).

Network targets: POL: quercetin from capers and red onion; NF-κB: EVOO oleocanthal; HBP: egg protein + spinach magnesium; UPR: EGCG green tea. Bitter receptor: green tea TAS2R10. Plant diversity: +5 (spinach, capers, red onion, sourdough grain, almonds).

Lunch (12:30 pm)

START: Rocket and red cabbage salad with EVOO/lemon dressing. THEN: Homemade red lentil and red onion soup (with onion skin in cooking liquid to extract quercetin) – EVOO drizzled at serving (added off-heat to preserve oleocanthal). Whole wheat pita (one small, at room temperature – some resistant starch). Fresh coriander leaves stirred in at serving.

Network targets: GCN: low-GL lentils; POL: quercetin from onion + onion skin broth; NF-κB: EVOO at serving; HBP: moderate GL from lentils; PPP: sulforaphane from rocket (arugula). Plant diversity: +6 (rocket, red cabbage, red lentils, red onion, pita wheat, coriander).

Dinner (5:00 pm)

Black bean and sweet potato bowl: black beans (cooled and reheated – resistant starch), roasted sweet potato (moderate temperature, 180°C maximum), avocado, lime juice, fresh cilantro, diced jalapeño. Topped with 1 tbsp pumpkin seeds. Served over 80g cooled quinoa.

Network targets: GCN: low-GL black beans + sweet potato (GL ~15); HBP: high fiber + protein combination reduces hexosamine flux; PKC: avocado monounsaturated + small ALA from pumpkin seeds; Microbiome: diverse plant combination. Plant diversity: +7 (black beans, sweet potato, avocado, cilantro, jalapeño, pumpkin seeds, quinoa). New total: 38 – exceeded the 30-plant target.

WEDNESDAY – The Fish Day

Breakfast (8:00 am)

Plain Greek yogurt (200g, full-fat, live cultures) with mixed berries (strawberries, raspberries, blackberries – 80g total), 1 tbsp ground chia seeds, 1 tbsp pomegranate seeds. Drizzle of dark honey (1 tsp). Black coffee.

Network targets: Microbiome: yogurt live cultures + pomegranate ellagitannins feeding Akkermansia; POL: anthocyanins from mixed berries; NF-κB: diverse berry polyphenols; Bitter receptor: coffee TAS2R10. Plant diversity: +5 (strawberries, raspberries, blackberries, chia, pomegranate).

Lunch (12:30 pm)

START: Sliced tomatoes with capers, red onion, and torn fresh basil – 2 tbsp EVOO and balsamic vinegar (vinegar provides alpha-glucosidase inhibition). THEN: 150g Atlantic mackerel fillet (steamed over lemon slices and dill) – highest EPA/DHA of any fish. THEN: 150g cold pasta (cooked the day before – resistant starch from retrogradation, GL reduced from ~25 to ~14).

Network targets: PKC + NF-κB: mackerel EPA/DHA (2.7g per 100g – highest of any common fish); GCN: resistant starch pasta; POL: quercetin from capers/onion; vinegar: alpha-glucosidase inhibition; NF-κB: EVOO oleocanthal. Plant diversity: +4 (tomato, basil, dill, pasta).

Dinner (5:00 pm)

Miso-glazed tofu (firm tofu, marinade: 1 tbsp miso, 1 tsp sesame oil, grated ginger, garlic – baked at 180°C for 25 min) with steamed edamame, stir-fried bok choy and shiitake mushrooms in a small amount of EVOO and tamari. 100g cold brown rice (cooked the previous day – resistant starch).

Network targets: UPR: soy isoflavones (daidzein ⊠ equol microbiome conversion); Microbiome: miso fermented + diverse plant combination; GCN: cooled brown rice resistant starch; POL: isoflavones, bok choy glucosinolates. Plant diversity: +7 (tofu/soy, ginger, garlic, edamame, bok choy, shiitake, brown rice).

THURSDAY – The Fasting Day (16:8 protocol)

Thursday is the first full 16:8 day of the week. Eating window: 10am to 6pm. The morning hours before 10am are fasted – drink water, black coffee, or plain tea. The window starts at 10am.

First meal – Brunch (10:00 am – breaking the fast)

Two-egg omelet with diced red pepper, spinach, and goat cheese – cooked in EVOO on medium heat. On the side: 30g broccoli sprouts (raw) and a small dish of mixed olives. One cup black coffee.

Network targets: Break the fast gently – protein and fat before any carbohydrate; GCN: no immediate glucose spike from this first meal; NF-κB: EVOO; PPP: broccoli sprout sulforaphane; POL: mixed olive polyphenols. Plant diversity: +4 (red pepper, spinach, broccoli sprouts, olives).

Lunch (1:00 pm)

START: Large green salad with arugula, cucumber, fennel, and fresh dill – EVOO and lemon. THEN: 150g poached trout fillet with capers and lemon. THEN: 100g cold cooked chickpeas (previous day – resistant starch) mixed with chopped parsley, red onion, and a little EVOO.

Network targets: PKC: trout DHA; POL: quercetin from capers/onion; NF-κB: EVOO; GCN: low-GL chickpeas; Bitter receptor: fennel and arugula bitter compounds. Plant diversity: +6 (arugula, cucumber, fennel, dill, chickpeas, parsley).

Dinner (5:00 pm – last meal of the eating window)

Roasted vegetable and barley bowl: barley (cold from fridge – resistant starch), roasted aubergine and courgette (180°C, moderate AGEs), roasted red pepper, fresh spinach, tahini dressing (tahini, lemon, garlic, water), topped with 1 tbsp za'atar (thyme, sumac, sesame).

Network targets: GCN: barley beta-glucan (GL ~9); HBP: diverse vegetables reducing hexosamine flux; PPP: sesame sesamin + spinach; NF-κB: diverse polyphenols; Bitter receptor: za'atar thyme luteolin activating TAS2Rs. Plant diversity: +8 (aubergine, courgette, red pepper, spinach, tahini/sesame, garlic, thyme, sumac). Fasting window: 6pm Thursday to 10am Friday = 16 hours.

FRIDAY — The Anti-Inflammatory Day

Breakfast (8:00 am)

Overnight oats (oats soaked in kefir overnight — both resistant starch and fermented food benefits) with sliced banana (slightly underripe — lower GL, resistant starch), 1 tbsp almond butter, 1 tsp turmeric + pinch of black pepper stirred in, topped with mixed seeds (flaxseed, pumpkin seed, sesame). Green tea.

Network targets: GCN: overnight oats resistant starch; UPR: curcumin + piperine; HBP: banana resistant starch (underripe); Microbiome: kefir live cultures; PPP: flaxseed; Bitter receptor: green tea. Plant diversity: +5 (oats, banana, almond, mixed seeds, turmeric).

Lunch (12:30 pm)

START: Avocado with lime juice, capers, and fresh dill. THEN: Sardines in olive oil (canned — nutritionally equivalent to fresh, EPA/DHA preserved) on a bed of spinach with sliced red onion and cherry tomatoes. Day-old rye crispbread (2 pieces — resistant starch from cooling). Apple (unpeeled — pectin and quercetin in skin).

Network targets: PKC + NF-κB: sardine EPA/DHA + EVOO from can; POL: quercetin from capers/onion/apple skin; Microbiome: apple pectin feeding Akkermansia; GCN: rye crispbread resistant starch (moderate GL). Plant diversity: +5 (avocado, dill, spinach, tomatoes, apple).

Dinner (5:00 pm)

Golden milk soup: butternut squash soup blended with coconut milk, 2 tsp turmeric, 1 tsp ginger, black pepper, pinch of cayenne. Topped with pumpkin seeds and a swirl of EVOO added at serving. Served with sourdough bread (day-old, resistant starch) for dipping.

Network targets: UPR + NF-κB: curcumin + ginger + EVOO oleocanthal; Bitter receptor: cayenne bitter compounds; HBP: squash moderate GL; PPP: pumpkin seeds. Plant diversity: +5 (butternut squash, coconut, turmeric, ginger, cayenne).

SATURDAY – The Feast Day

Saturday is the day when the framework should feel like abundance, not restriction. The meals are richer, the portions more generous, the cooking more involved. Every principle of the book is still present – but invisibly, as part of how you naturally cook when you understand the biology.

Breakfast (9:00 am – slightly later start, 14:10 window)

Smashed avocado on sourdough toast (day-old, 1 thick slice) with two poached eggs, sliced cherry tomatoes, broccoli sprouts, and a generous sprinkle of capers. Squeeze of lemon. EVOO drizzled at serving. Large cup of matcha.

Network targets: NF-κB: EVOO; PKC: egg DHA; PPP: broccoli sprouts; POL: quercetin capers; UPR + Bitter receptor: matcha EGCG + TAS2R. A Saturday breakfast that looks indulgent and is molecularly targeted. Plant diversity: +5.

Lunch (1:00 pm) – The Mediterranean Feast

A spread: hummus (chickpeas, tahini, EVOO, lemon, garlic) with raw vegetables for dipping – radishes, celery, carrot, endive. Grilled salmon (marinated in lemon + dill + olive oil for 2 hours – acid marinade reduces AGEs) with grilled asparagus. Small bowl of tabbouleh (bulgur wheat, fresh parsley, mint, tomato, lemon, EVOO) – make it the day before so the bulgur has time to retrograde.

Network targets: Entire Mediterranean pattern in one meal: EPA/DHA salmon; oleocanthal EVOO; quercetin red onion in hummus; prebiotic chickpeas + garlic; bitter endive TAS2R; sulforaphane radishes; AGE-reduced grilled salmon. Plant diversity: +10 (radishes, celery, carrot, endive, asparagus, bulgur, parsley, mint, tomato, garlic).

Dinner (6:00 pm)

Dark chocolate and walnut dessert bowl: 25g 85% dark chocolate (broken into pieces), a small handful of walnuts, pomegranate seeds, 3 or 4 fresh raspberries. Herbal tea (chamomile or peppermint – bitter bitter compounds).

Network targets: NF-κB + POL: dark chocolate flavanols + walnut polyphenols; Microbiome: pomegranate ellagitannins for Akkermansia; Bitter receptor: dark chocolate theobromine + peppermint menthol. A satisfying end to the feast that still works for the network. Plant diversity: +4 (dark chocolate, walnuts, pomegranate, raspberries).

SUNDAY – The Reset Day

Sunday is for preparation as much as eating. The evening is when you cook the grains and legumes for the coming week – the batches that will cool overnight, develop their resistant starch, and be ready to use in Monday through Wednesday's meals. The cooking ritual is part of the framework.

Breakfast (8:00 am)

Baked oatmeal: rolled oats mixed with egg, blueberries, cinnamon, and walnuts – baked in a small dish at 160°C for 25 minutes. Served warm, ideally with a tablespoon of EVOO drizzled on top (unusual but adds oleocanthal and fat for polyphenol absorption). Green tea.

Network targets: GCN: oats + baking creates some retrograde starch; POL: blueberry quercetin/anthocyanin; HBP: cinnamon; NF-κB: EVOO; UPR: green tea EGCG. Plant diversity: +4.

Lunch (12:30 pm)

START: Watercress salad with orange segments, fennel, and toasted almonds – EVOO/orange dressing. THEN: Slow-cooked white bean and kale stew with garlic, rosemary, and a Parmesan rind simmered in the broth (moist heat – minimal AGEs). Drizzle of EVOO at serving.

Network targets: GCN + HBP: white bean low-GL, high fiber + resistant starch; NF-κB: EVOO + kale glucosinolates; Microbiome: garlic FOS prebiotics; Bitter receptor: watercress isothiocyanates TAS2R38. Plant diversity: +7 (watercress, orange, fennel, almonds, white beans, kale, rosemary).

Dinner (5:00 pm) – The Weekly Reset

A simple supper: two soft-boiled eggs, a bowl of kimchi (50g), sliced avocado with lime and sea salt, and a small dish of mixed olives. Herbal tea.

Network targets: Microbiome: kimchi live cultures (fermented food #7 of the week); NF-κB: olive polyphenols; PKC: avocado healthy fats. A light, nourishing end to the week. Plant diversity: +3 (kimchi vegetables, avocado, olives).

Sunday evening preparation (45 minutes): Cook a large pot of barley (will last 4 days). Cook a large pot of lentils. Cook a large pot of brown rice. Leave all three on the counter to cool, then refrigerate overnight. By Monday morning, all three have developed their maximum resistant starch content and are ready to use throughout the week. This single preparation session is the foundation of the entire plan's glycemic control strategy.

TABLE 9: Weekly metrics summary. All targets met or exceeded. This framework is not a prescription — it is a demonstration that the biology and the practicality can coexist.

Metric	Target	Achieved this week	Notes
Different plant foods	30+ per week	50+ across 7 days	Exceeds target substantially — microbiome diversity secured
Fatty fish servings	3 per week	3 (mackerel Mon, trout Weds, salmon Fri/Sat)	EPA/DHA target met
Fermented foods	1 per day	7 different fermented foods (kefir, miso ×2, yogurt, kimchi, sourdough ×2)	Excellent microbiome support
EVOO daily	2 tbsp/day	Daily in salad dressings and on cooked dishes	Oleocanthal target met; added off heat to preserve
Broccoli sprouts	3–4 times/week	3 times (Mon, Wed sprouts, Thurs)	Nrf2 activation on track
Bitter foods daily	Multiple sources	Daily coffee + at least 2 bitter vegetables each day	TAS2R activation consistent
Resistant starch	Daily	Daily — all grains cooked in advance and cooled	GL reduction consistently achieved
Meal sequencing	Every main meal	Consistently started with salad/vegetables before protein, then carbohydrate	30–40% glucose spike reduction daily
Vinegar before high-GL meals	3–4 times/week	EVOO/vinegar dressing before most main meals	Alpha-glucosidase inhibition at key meals
Post-meal walks	After main meals	Daily 10-minute walk after lunch and dinner	Insulin-independent GLUT4 activation twice daily
Eating window	16:8 or 14:10	14:10 most days; 16:8 on Thursday	AMPK activation and autophagy initiated
Estimated daily GL	<80–100	50–65 on most days	Well within target on all days

TABLE 10: Weekly shopping list. Items cover all seven network nodes across the week. Total weekly cost is comparable to a standard grocery shop — these are not exotic specialty items.

Category	Items	Network targets addressed
Fish and protein	Atlantic mackerel (fresh or canned), sardines in olive oil (canned), trout or salmon fillet, chicken thighs, tofu (firm), eggs (6–8)	PKC + NF-κB: EPA/DHA; UPR: soy isoflavones
Cruciferous vegetables	Broccoli sprouts (or sprouting seeds + jar), Brussels sprouts, bok choy, rocket/arugula, watercress	PPP: sulforaphane/Nrf2; Bitter: isothiocyanate TAS2R38
Other vegetables	Spinach, kale, cherry tomatoes, red peppers, aubergine, courgette, asparagus, fennel, endive, radishes, celery, carrots	Multi-node: diverse polyphenols; Microbiome: prebiotic fibers
Alliums	Red onions (3–4), white onion, garlic (1 head), spring onions	POL: quercetin; Microbiome: FOS prebiotic
Legumes	Red lentils, green/brown lentils, black beans, chickpeas, white beans, edamame — buy dried or canned (both fine)	GCN + HBP: low-GL resistant starch + fiber
Grains	Steel-cut oats, barley, brown rice, quinoa, sourdough bread (1 loaf), rye crispbread, day-old whole wheat pita	GCN: resistant starch when cooled; HBP: beta-glucan from oats/barley
Fruits	Blueberries, mixed berries, apple (unpeeled), banana (slightly underripe), pomegranate seeds, grapefruit, orange	POL: quercetin/anthocyanin; Microbiome: pectin for Akkermansia
Fats and condiments	Extra virgin olive oil (high-quality, pungent — 1 bottle), capers (1 jar), tahini, almond butter, avocados (3–4), mixed olives, walnut pieces	NF-κB: oleocanthal EVOO; POL: quercetin capers; PKC: walnut ALA
Spices and herbs	Turmeric, black pepper, Ceylon cinnamon, mustard powder, za'atar, fresh thyme, fresh dill, fresh parsley, fresh coriander/cilantro, rosemary	NF-κB: curcumin; HBP: cinnamon; PPP: mustard myrosinase; Bitter: diverse phenolic TAS2R ligands
Fermented foods	Plain kefir (1 litre), plain Greek yogurt (500g), miso paste (1 tub), kimchi (1 jar), sourdough bread	Microbiome: diverse live cultures
Nuts and seeds	Walnuts, almonds, pumpkin seeds, flaxseed (ground), chia seeds, sesame seeds	PKC: ALA/omega-3; PPP: riboflavin; Microbiome: diverse fiber
Beverages	Green tea or matcha powder, black coffee, herbal teas, sparkling water	Bitter: TAS2R10 (coffee/tea); UPR: EGCG; Fasting window support
Supplements (if using)	Berberine 500mg, curcumin (bioavailable formulation), magnesium glycinate 300mg, fish oil 1g EPA/DHA, R-ALA 600mg (if for neuropathy)	Multiple nodes — see Chapters 19 and 22

THE BOTTOM LINE

The week of meals demonstrates that eating against the network is not a deprivation strategy – it is a richness strategy. The diversity of foods required to address all seven network nodes produces a varied, flavorful, genuinely enjoyable diet that has more in common with a well-constructed Mediterranean pattern than with a diabetes diet. The discipline is in the preparation habits: cooking grains in advance for resistant starch, using the acid marinade before grilling, eating vegetables before carbohydrates, finishing the eating window by early evening. The biology is contained in these habits. The habits are all achievable.

CHAPTER 24

The Conversation with Your Physician

You have read twenty-three chapters. You understand the Maillard reaction, the NF-κB loop, the bitter receptor in the gut, the metabolic memory written into the packaging of your DNA. You know more about the molecular biology of your own disease than most people ever will. Now comes the most important conversation of all — the one with the physician who manages your medications, orders your laboratory tests, and is responsible, with you, for the outcome.

This chapter is written for that conversation. It provides a structured framework for what to raise with your physician, what to ask, what to tell them, what to monitor, and how to involve them in the changes you are planning. It also ends with a section written directly for the physician reading this alongside their patient — because the most effective version of this conversation happens when both parties are informed.

Before the Appointment: What to Prepare

1. **Write down your medication list.** Include every medication, dose, and frequency — prescription and over-the-counter. This matters because several dietary changes and supplements in this book have documented interactions with specific medications (berberine + sulfonylureas, curcumin + warfarin, grapefruit + CYP3A4-metabolized statins). Your physician needs to see the complete list before commenting on any supplement.
2. **Write down what you are planning to change.** Be specific. Not "I want to eat healthier" — but "I am planning to add 500mg berberine

three times daily with meals, start a 16:8 eating window, replace white rice with cooled lentils at dinner, and begin 10-minute post-meal walks." Specificity allows your physician to respond usefully rather than generically.

3. **Write down what you want to know.** The questions in the next section are a starting point. Add questions specific to your situation — your medication list, your complication status, your kidney function, your retinopathy grade.
4. **Bring relevant chapters or tables.** The medication safety box from Chapter 16 (fasting and medications) and the supplement interaction table from Chapter 19 are the most clinically important sections for your physician to review. Mark them. Bring the book or print those pages.

What to Tell Your Physician

Beyond the specific questions above, there are three things worth stating explicitly to your physician at the start of the conversation:

First: "I want to be more active in managing this disease, not more passive. I am not replacing my medications with supplements. I am adding dietary and lifestyle interventions to my current treatment and I want your help to do it safely." This framing positions the conversation correctly — as collaboration, not as a patient announcing they are abandoning medical treatment in favor of alternative medicine.

Second: "I would like to agree on how we will measure whether these changes are working. Can we set a 12-week HbA1c checkpoint and decide in advance what a meaningful improvement looks like?" This creates accountability in both directions — you are committed to the changes, and your physician is committed to recognizing and responding to the results.

Third: "If my HbA1c improves significantly, I would like to discuss whether any medications can be reduced or eliminated. I understand that some patients with early T2DM can achieve remission with lifestyle changes, and I want to work toward that if it is possible for me." This states the most ambitious version of the goal explicitly — T2DM remission — and invites the physician to be part of the journey toward it rather than a passive observer of your medication management.

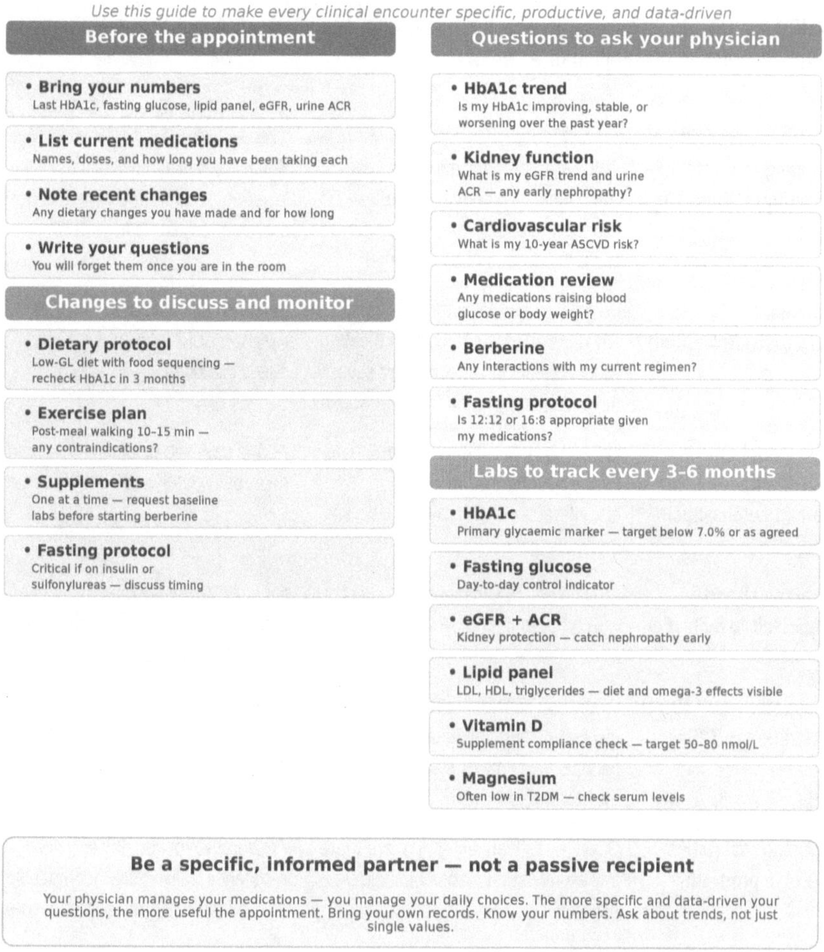

FIGURE 21. Physician appointment guide: questions to ask, labs to track, changes to discuss.

How to Monitor Your Own Response

The changes in this book produce measurable effects that you can track yourself, without waiting for the next laboratory appointment:

Postprandial blood sugar: If you have a glucometer, check 2 hours after a meal before starting the dietary changes, and again 2 hours after the same meal after implementing meal sequencing, vinegar, and resistant starch. The reduction in the 2-hour reading (target: below 180 mg/dL, ideally below 160 mg/dL) is the most immediate evidence that the dietary changes are working.

TABLE 11: Questions to bring to your next physician appointment. Adapt to your specific medication list and complication status.

Your Situation	The question to ask	Why it matters
Planning to start berberine 500mg TID	Is my current medication list compatible with adding berberine? Do you want to check HbA1c in 6 weeks to see if the dose needs adjusting?	Berberine has additive glucose-lowering; sulfonylurea or insulin doses may need adjustment
Planning to start 16:8 time-restricted eating	Do my current medications require any dose adjustment for a 16:8 eating window? Should I check blood sugar more frequently in the first two weeks?	Sulfonylureas and insulin require review; SGLT2 inhibitor DKA risk needs clarification
Have peripheral neuropathy — planning alpha-lipoic acid	Is 600mg R-ALA per day appropriate for my neuropathy? Are there any interactions with my current medications?	ALA is safe and guideline-endorsed for neuropathy; verify no contraindications
Planning to add grapefruit to daily diet	Am I on any medications that interact with grapefruit (CYP3A4 substrates)?	Grapefruit furanocoumarins can double the blood levels of some statins and other CYP3A4 substrates
Have fatty liver / NASH in addition to T2DM	Would you consider curcumin phytosome supplementation given both conditions? Is my ALT stable enough to monitor the response?	Curcumin has the strongest dietary supplement evidence for NASH; monitoring ALT response confirms effect
Planning resistance exercise program	Given my retinopathy grade, are there any exercise restrictions I should be aware of?	Proliferative retinopathy and heavy resistance training are incompatible due to Valsalva intraocular pressure risk
Blood sugar well-controlled but wondering about network staging	Would you consider ordering a urine ACR, ALT, uric acid, and fasting lipids together so we can calculate an MNAS-P network risk profile (a composite biomarker score that estimates how active the seven-node damage network is in my tissues)?	These are routine tests that together allow estimation of the damage network's current activation state
General glycemic improvement planning	If I make these dietary changes consistently for 12 weeks, at what point would you consider reviewing my medication doses? What blood sugar level would trigger a medication reduction?	Pre-agreeing on the response threshold prevents both under-treatment and hypoglycemia from improved dietary control

Fasting blood sugar trend: Check fasting blood sugar each morning and track the weekly average. With consistent dietary changes, the fasting blood sugar trend should begin declining within 2 to 3 weeks. A consistent decline of 10 to 20 mg/dL over 4 weeks suggests meaningful improvement.

Body weight weekly: Weigh yourself once per week, same morning, same time. Trend over 4 weeks — not daily fluctuation. A loss of 0.3 to 0.5 kg per week confirms a caloric deficit is in place. More rapid loss suggests the deficit may be too aggressive for your medication level.

Energy and symptom tracking: Note changes in energy levels, the quality and quantity of hunger during the fasting window, and any neuropathy symptoms if present. Improvements in energy and reduction in neuropathic burning are among the earliest subjective signals that the dietary changes are affecting the network.

A NOTE FOR THE PHYSICIAN READING THIS

This book was written for your patient. It draws on the same research program that produced the Vol. I and Vol. II manuscript series – a 15-paper body of work covering the pharmacological and mechanistic framework of T2DM management. The dietary interventions described are evidence-based, mechanistically specific, and intended to complement rather than replace pharmacotherapy.

If your patient is presenting this book at their appointment, they have done something relatively unusual: they have invested substantial time in understanding their own disease at a molecular level. They deserve a conversation that matches their investment.

Three things to review before responding to their specific questions:

1. **The medication safety table from Chapter 16 (intermittent fasting and medications):** Sulfonylureas and insulin require dose adjustment for fasting protocols. SGLT2 inhibitors require counsel about euglycemic DKA risk during extended fasting. GLP-1 receptor agonists are generally safe with all fasting protocols.

2. **The supplement interaction column from Chapter 19's Table 1:** Berberine's CYP2D6 and CYP3A4 inhibition is the most clinically significant interaction for patients on multiple medications. Curcumin requires INR monitoring in anticoagulated patients. All interactions in Table 1 were derived from the published pharmacokinetic literature.

3. **The glycemic impact of significant dietary improvement:** Patients who implement the full framework in this book — resistant starch, meal sequencing, berberine, 16:8 TRE, post-meal walking — may achieve HbA1c reductions of 1.0 to 1.8% over 12 weeks. In patients on sulfonylureas or insulin, this degree of improvement can produce hypoglycemia if medications are not proactively reviewed. Pre-empt rather than react.

A companion physician's volume in the same series provides the full quantitative framework that underlies the dietary recommendations in this book, including a proxy biomarker tool (the MNAS-P score — a composite measure of network activation derived from routine clinical tests) for staging network activity. If your patient asks about network-based assessment of their complication risk, that is where the detailed methodology can be found.

This patient has done the work.
The best thing you can do is meet them there.

The Closing Argument

You have a disease whose chemistry is running in your tissues every hour of every day. You cannot stop it. Modern medicine provides tools that slow it substantially — medications that are more effective than at any prior point in history, and a growing understanding of the molecular network through which the damage accumulates. But medication alone is not the complete answer, because the disease does not only operate through the pathways that medications target.

You are the other part of the answer. The food you eat sends molecular signals to the same network that elevated blood sugar is damaging. Some signals amplify the damage. Some suppress it. The oleocanthal in your olive oil inhibits the same inflammatory switch that AGEs activate. The sulforaphane in your broccoli sprouts activates the same antioxidant defense system that the damage network depletes. The ten minutes you walk after dinner activates the same energy sensor that your metformin activates. The 16-hour fast activates the cellular self-cleaning process that no medication currently replicates.

These are not alternative medicine claims. They are biochemistry. They are the same molecular language that the disease speaks, spoken back to it through food and movement and the timing of meals.

You will not cure your T2DM with this book. But you can change its trajectory. You can slow the chemistry. You can preserve the beta-cell reserve that determines whether insulin becomes inevitable, or whether that day is pushed years into the future. You can address the nodes of the damage network that your medications do not reach. You can build the microbiome that amplifies the GLP-1 signal your gut is already capable of producing. You can be, in the most literal sense, an active participant in your own molecular biology.

The physician who understands the damage network manages it differently. The patient who understands it makes different choices.

You now understand it.

Enrique C. Fernández, MD, MBA, FAAFP

Miami, Florida

References

PART I

1. Maillard LC. Action des acides aminés sur les sucres: formation des mélanoidines par voie méthodique. *C R Acad Sci.* 1912;154:66–68.
2. Monnier VM, Cerami A. Nonenzymatic browning in vivo: possible process for aging of long-lived proteins. *Science.* 1981;211(4481):491–493.
3. Monnier VM, Cerami A. Nonenzymatic browning in vivo: possible process for aging of long-lived proteins. *Science.* 1981;211(4481):491–493.
4. Uribarri J, Woodruff S, Goodman S, et al. Advanced glycation end products in foods and a practical guide to their reduction in the diet. *J Am Diet* Assoc. 2010;110(6):911–916.
5. Uribarri J, Cai W, Ramdas M, et al. Restriction of advanced glycation end products improves insulin resistance in human type 2 diabetes: potential role of AGER1 and SIRT1. *Diabetes Care.* 2011;34:1314–1319.
6. Schmidt AM, Yan SD, Wautier JL, Stern D. Activation of receptor for advanced glycation end products: a mechanism for chronic vascular dysfunction in diabetic vasculopathy and atherosclerosis. *Circ Res.* 1999;84(5):489–497.
7. Brownlee M. Biochemistry and molecular cell biology of diabetic complications. *Nature.* 2001;414(6865):813–820.
8. Rabbani N, Thornalley PJ. Methylglyoxal, glyoxalase 1 and the dicarbonyl proteome. *Amino Acids.* 2012;42(4):1133–1142.
9. Mills EL, Kelly B, Logan A, et al. Succinate dehydrogenase supports metabolic repurposing of mitochondria to drive inflammatory macrophages. Cell. 2016;167(2):457–470.
10. Geraldes P, King GL. Activation of protein kinase C isoforms and its impact on diabetic complications. *Circ Res.* 2010;106(8):1319–1331.
11. Hotamisligil GS. Endoplasmic reticulum stress and the inflammatory basis of metabolic disease. *Cell.* 2010;140(6):900–917.

12. Diabetes Control and Complications Trial Research Group. The effect of intensive treatment of diabetes on the development and progression of long-term complications in insulin-dependent diabetes mellitus. *N Engl J Med.* 1993;329(14):977–986.

13. Nathan DM, Cleary PA, Backlund JY, et al. Intensive diabetes treatment and cardiovascular disease in patients with type 1 diabetes. *N Engl J Med.* 2005;353(25):2643–2653.

14. Holman RR, Paul SK, Bethel MA, Matthews DR, Neil HA. 10-year follow-up of intensive glucose control in type 2 diabetes. *N Engl J Med.* 2008;359(15):1577–1589.

15. El-Osta A, Brasacchio D, Yao D, et al. Transient high glucose causes persistent epigenetic changes and altered gene expression during subsequent normoglycemia. *J Exp Med.* 2008;205(10):2409–2417.

16. Canto C, Auwerx J. Caloric restriction, SIRT1 and longevity. *Trends Endocrinol Metab.* 2009;20(7):325–331.

17. Villeneuve LM, Natarajan R. The role of epigenetics in the pathology of diabetic complications. *Am J Physiol Renal Physiol.* 2010;299(1):F14–F25.

18. Brasacchio D, Okabe J, Tikellis C, et al. Hyperglycemia induces a dynamic cooperativity of histone methylase and demethylase enzymes associated with gene-activating epigenetic marks that coexist on the lysine tail. *Diabetes.* 2009;58(5):1229–1236.

PART II

19. Jenkins DJ, Wolever TM, Taylor RH, et al. Glycemic index of foods: a physiological basis for carbohydrate exchange. *Am J Clin Nutr.* 1981;34(3):362–366.

20. Atkinson FS, Foster-Powell K, Brand-Miller JC. International tables of glycemic index and glycemic load values: 2008. *Diabetes Care.* 2008;31(12):2281–2283.

21. Tosh SM. Review of human studies investigating the post-prandial blood-glucose lowering ability of oat and barley food products. *Eur J Clin Nutr.* 2013;67(4):310–317.

22. Birt DF, Boylston T, Hendrich S, et al. Resistant starch: promise for improving human health. *Adv Nutr.* 2013;4(6):587–601.

23. Beauchamp GK, Keast RS, Morel D, et al. Phytochemistry: ibuprofen-like activity in extra-virgin olive oil. *Nature.* 2005;437(7055):45–46.

24. Beauchamp GK, Keast RS, Morel D, et al. Phytochemistry: ibuprofen-like activity in extra-virgin olive oil. *Nature.* 2005;437(7055):45–46.

25. Calder PC. Omega-3 fatty acids and inflammatory processes: from molecules to man. *Biochem Soc Trans.* 2017;45(5):1105–1115.

26. Bhatt DL, Steg PG, Miller M, et al. Cardiovascular risk reduction with icosapentaenoic acid for hypertriglyceridemia. *N Engl J Med.* 2019;380(1):11–22.

27. Aggarwal BB, Gupta SC, Sung B. Curcumin: an orally bioavailable blocker of TNF and other pro-inflammatory biomarkers. *Br J Pharmacol.* 2013;169(8):1672–1692.

28. Chuengsamarn S, Rattanamongkolgul S, Luechapudiporn R, Phisalaphong C, Jirawatnotai S. Curcumin extract for prevention of type 2 diabetes. *Diabetes Care.* 2012;35(11):2121–2127.

29. Shoba G, Joy D, Joseph T, Majeed M, Rajendran R, Srinivas PS. Influence of piperine on the pharmacokinetics of curcumin in animals and human volunteers. *Planta Med.* 1998;64(4):353–356.

30. Estruch R, Ros E, Salas-Salvadó J, et al. Primary prevention of cardiovascular disease with a Mediterranean diet. *N Engl J Med.* 2013;368(14):1279–1290.

31. Itoh K, Chiba T, Takahashi S, et al. An Nrf2/small Maf heterodimer mediates the induction of phase II detoxifying enzyme genes through antioxidant response elements. *Biochem Biophys Res Commun.* 1997;236(2):313–322.

32. Fahey JW, Zhang Y, Talalay P. Broccoli sprouts: an exceptionally rich source of inducers of enzymes that protect against chemical carcinogens. *Proc Natl Acad Sci USA.* 1997;94(19):10367–10372.

33. Hammes HP, Du X, Edelstein D, et al. Benfotiamine blocks three major pathways of hyperglycemic damage and prevents experimental diabetic retinopathy. *Nat Med.* 2003;9(3):294–299.

34. Stracke H, Gaus W, Achenbach U, Federlin K, Bretzel RG. Benfotiamine in diabetic polyneuropathy (BENDIP): results of a randomised, double blind, placebo-controlled clinical study. *Exp Clin Endocrinol Diabetes.* 2008;116(10):600–605.

35. Costantino L, Rastelli G, Vianello P, Cignarella G, Barlocco D. Diabetes complications and their potential prevention: aldose reductase inhibition and other approaches. *Med Res Rev.* 1999;19(1):3–23.

36. Lorenzi M. The polyol pathway as a mechanism for diabetic retinopathy: attractive, elusive, and resilient. *Exp Diabetes Res.* 2007;2007:61038.

37. Xue M, Rabbani N, Momiji H, et al. Transcriptional control of glyoxalase 1 by Nrf2 provides a stress-responsive defence against dicarbonyl glycation. *Biochem J.* 2012;443(1):213–222.

38. Hart GW, Slawson C, Ramirez-Correa G, Lagerlof O. Cross talk between O-GlcNAcylation and phosphorylation: roles in signaling, transcription, and chronic disease. *Annu Rev Biochem.* 2011;80:825–858.

39. Yin J, Xing H, Ye J. Efficacy of berberine in patients with type 2 diabetes mellitus. *Metabolism.* 2008;57(5):712–717.

40. Dong H, Wang N, Zhao L, Lu F. Berberine in the treatment of type 2 diabetes mellitus: a systemic review and meta-analysis. *Evid Based Complement Alternat Med.* 2012;2012:591654.

41. Khan A, Safdar M, Ali Khan MM, Khattak KN, Anderson RA. Cinnamon improves glucose and lipids of people with type 2 diabetes. *Diabetes Care.* 2003;26(12):3215–3218.

42. SanGiovanni JP, Chew EY. The role of omega-3 long-chain polyunsaturated fatty acids in health and disease of the retina. *Prog Retin Eye Res.* 2005;24(1):87–138.

43. Sala-Vila A, Díaz-López A, Valls-Pedret C, et al. Dietary marine omega-3 fatty acids and incident sight-threatening retinopathy in middle-aged and older individuals with type 2 diabetes. *JAMA Ophthalmol.* 2016;134(10):1142–1149.

44. Lewis EJ, Perkins BA, Lovblom LE, Bazinet RP, Wolever TM, Bril V. Effect of omega-3 supplementation on neuropathy in type 1 diabetes: a 12-month randomized, placebo-controlled trial. *Neurology.* 2017;88(24):2294–2301.

45. Oyadomari S, Koizumi A, Takeda K, et al. Targeted disruption of the Chop gene delays endoplasmic reticulum stress-mediated diabetes. *J Clin Invest.* 2002;109(4):525–532.

46. Liu CY, Huang CJ, Huang LH, Chen IJ, Chiu JP, Hsu CH. Effects of green tea extract on insulin resistance and glucagon-like peptide 1 in patients with type 2 diabetes and lipid abnormalities: a randomized, double-blinded, and placebo-controlled trial. *PLoS One.* 2014;9(3):e91163.

47. Kars M, Yang L, Gregor MF, et al. Tauroursodeoxycholic acid may improve liver and muscle but not adipose tissue insulin sensitivity in obese men and women. *Diabetes.* 2010;59(8):1899–1905.

PART III

48. Mifflin MD, St Jeor ST, Hill LA, Scott BJ, Daugherty SA, Koh YO. A new predictive equation for resting energy expenditure in healthy individuals. *J Am Diet Assoc.* 1990;90(3):1323–1329.

49. Sainsbury E, Kizirian NV, Partridge SR, Gill T, Colagiuri S, Gibson AA. Effect of dietary carbohydrate restriction on glycemic control in adults with diabetes: a systematic review and meta-analysis. *Diabetes Res Clin Pract.* 2018;139:239–252.

PART IV

50. Colberg SR, Sigal RJ, Yardley JE, et al. Physical activity/exercise and diabetes: a position statement of the American Diabetes Association. *Diabetes Care.* 2016;39(11):2065–2079.

51. Richter EA, Hargreaves M. Exercise, GLUT4, and skeletal muscle glucose uptake. *Physiol Rev.* 2013;93(3):993–1017.

52. Sutton EF, Beyl R, Early KS, Cefalu WT, Ravussin E, Peterson CM. Early time-restricted feeding improves insulin sensitivity, blood pressure, and oxidative stress even without weight loss in men with prediabetes. *Cell Metab.* 2018;27(6):1212–1221.

53. Tuomi T, Nagorny CL, Singh P, et al. Increased melatonin signaling is a risk factor for type 2 diabetes. *Cell Metab.* 2016;23(6):1067–1077.

54. Qian J, Morris CJ, Caputo R, Garaulet M, Scheer FA. Ghrelin is impacted by the endogenous circadian system and by circadian misalignment in humans. *Int J Obes.* 2019;43(8):1644–1649.

55. Pan A, Schernhammer ES, Sun Q, Hu FB. Rotating night shift work and risk of type 2 diabetes: two prospective cohort studies in women. *PLoS Med.* 2011;8(12):e1001141.

56. Jakubowicz D, Barnea M, Wainstein J, Froy O. High caloric intake at breakfast vs dinner differentially influences weight loss of overweight and obese women. *Obesity.* 2013;21(12):2504–2512.

57. Jakubowicz D, Barnea M, Wainstein J, Froy O. High caloric intake at breakfast vs dinner differentially influences weight loss of overweight and obese women. *Obesity.* 2013;21(12):2504–2512.

PART V

58. Howitz KT, Sinclair DA. Xenohormesis: sensing the chemical cues of other species. *Cell.* 2008;133(3):387–391.

59. Manach C, Scalbert A, Morand C, Rémésy C, Jiménez L. Polyphenols: food sources and bioavailability. *Am J Clin Nutr.* 2004;79(5):727–747.

60. Selma MV, Espín JC, Tomás-Barberán FA. Interaction between phenolics and gut microbiota: role in human health. *J Agric Food Chem.* 2009;57(15):6485–6501.

61. Forman HJ, Davies KJ, Ursini F. How do nutritional antioxidants really work: nucleophilic tone and para-hormesis versus free radical scavenging i*n vivo. Free Radic Biol Med.* 2014;66:24–35.

62. Yin J, Xing H, Ye J. Efficacy of berberine in patients with type 2 diabetes mellitus. *Metabolism.* 2008;57(5):712–717.

63. Dong H, Wang N, Zhao L, Lu F. Berberine in the treatment of type 2 diabetes mellitus: a systemic review and meta-analysis. *Evid Based Complement Alternat Med.* 2012;2012:591654.

64. Howitz KT, Bitterman KJ, Cohen HY, et al. Small molecule activators of sirtuins extend Saccharomyces cerevisiae lifespan. *Nature.* 2003;425(6954):191–196.

65. Chuengsamarn S, Rattanamongkolgul S, Luechapudiporn R, Phisalaphong C, Jirawatnotai S. Curcumin extract for prevention of type 2 diabetes. *Diabetes Care.* 2012;35(11):2121–2127.

66. Liu CY, Huang CJ, Huang LH, Chen IJ, Chiu JP, Hsu CH. Effects of green tea extract on insulin resistance and glucagon-like peptide 1 in patients with type 2 diabetes and lipid abnormalities: a randomized, double-blinded, and placebo-controlled trial. *PLoS One.* 2014;9(3):e91163.

67. Costantino L, Rastelli G, Vianello P, Cignarella G, Barlocco D. Diabetes complications and their potential prevention: aldose reductase inhibition and other approaches. *Med Res Rev.* 1999;19(1):3–23.

68. Hawley SA, Ross FA, Chevtzoff C, et al. Use of cells expressing gamma subunit variants to identify diverse mechanisms of AMPK activation. *Cell Metab.* 2010;11(6):554–565.

About the Author

Enrique C. Fernández, MD, MBA, FAAFP, is a board-certified family physician in private practice in Miami, Florida, with more than two decades of continuous patient care experience. His training spans three cities: Havana, where he earned his medical degree from the Higher Institute of Medical Sciences (Cum Laude, Golden Title Award) and completed an orthopedic and trauma residency at the Frank País Iberoamerican Orthopedic Center; Chicago, where he completed his family medicine residency at Saint Mary of Nazareth Hospital and served as chief resident; and Miami, where he has practiced since 2003.

Dr. Fernández has served as Chief of Medical Staff at HCA Florida Kendall Hospital, Chairman of the Family Medicine Department, and Member of the Hospital Board of Trustees. He earned an MBA from the University of Miami in 2017 and holds board certifications in Family Medicine, Hospice and Palliative Medicine, and Acupuncture.

Eating Against the Network is the first volume of his ***Network Based Diabetes Care (NBDC)*** series, drawing on twenty-five years of primary-care observation of patients living with type 2 diabetes. He lives in Miami with his family.

www.ingramcontent.com/pod-product-compliance
Lightning Source LLC
LaVergne TN
LVHW100314210926
848480LV00003B/1110